Histoplasmosis - A Comprehensive Study of Epidemiology, Pathogenesis, Diagnosis, and Treatment

Edited by Elena Dantes and Elena Dumea

Published in London, United Kingdom

Histoplasmosis - A Comprehensive Study of Epidemiology, Pathogenesis, Diagnosis, and Treatment
http://dx.doi.org/10.5772/intechopen.104142
Edited by Elena Dantes and Elena Dumea

Contributors
Filipa Sousa, Domingos Ferreira, Salette Reis, Paulo Costa, Israel Kiiza Njovu, Pauline Petra Nalumaga, Kennedy Kasaaza, Edwin Nuwagira, Joel Bazira, Lucas Ampaire, Herbert Itabangi, Monica Marc, Diana Manolescu, Estera Boeriu, Ana Adriana Trusculescu, Milena Adina Man, Doina Adina Todea, Nicoleta Ștefania Motoc, Ruxandra-Mioara Rajnoveanu, Nela Daniela Efrim, Elena Dumea, Roxana Carmen Cernat, Elena Dantes, Roxana-Carmen Cernat

First published in London, United Kingdom, 2023 by IntechOpen
IntechOpen is the global imprint of INTECHOPEN LIMITED, registered in England and Wales, registration number: 11086078, 5 Princes Gate Court, London, SW7 2QJ, United Kingdom
Printed in Croatia

British Library Cataloguing-in-Publication Data
A catalogue record for this book is available from the British Library

Additional hard and PDF copies can be obtained from orders@intechopen.com

Histoplasmosis - A Comprehensive Study of Epidemiology, Pathogenesis, Diagnosis, and Treatment
Edited by Elena Dantes and Elena Dumea
p. cm.

This title is part of the Infectious Diseases Book Series, Volume 24
Topic: Fungal Infectious Diseases
Series Editor: Alfonso J. Rodriguez-Morales
Topic Editor: Yuping Ran

Print ISBN 978-1-83768-661-2
Online ISBN 978-1-83768-662-9
eBook (PDF) ISBN 978-1-83768-663-6
ISSN 2631-6188

IntechOpen Book Series
Infectious Diseases
Volume 24

Aims and Scope of the Series

This series will provide a comprehensive overview of recent research trends in various Infectious Diseases (as per the most recent Baltimore classification). Topics will include general overviews of infections, immunopathology, diagnosis, treatment, epidemiology, etiology, and current clinical recommendations for managing infectious diseases. Ongoing issues, recent advances, and future diagnostic approaches and therapeutic strategies will also be discussed. This book series will focus on various aspects and properties of infectious diseases whose deep understanding is essential for safeguarding the human race from losing resources and economies due to pathogens.

Meet the Series Editor

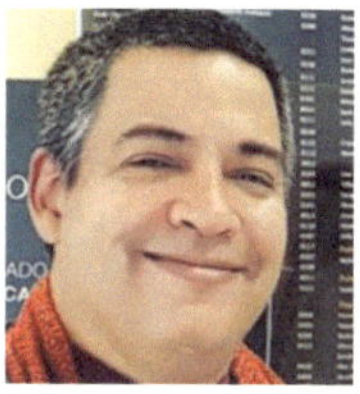

Dr. Rodriguez-Morales is an expert in tropical and emerging diseases, particularly zoonotic and vector-borne diseases (notably arboviral diseases), and more recently COVID-19 and Monkeypox. He is the president of the Publications and Research Committee of the Pan-American Infectious Diseases Association (API), as well as the president of the Colombian Association of Infectious Diseases (ACIN). He is a member of the Committee on Tropical Medicine, Zoonoses, and Travel Medicine of ACIN. Dr. Rodriguez-Morales is a vice-president of the Latin American Society for Travel Medicine (SLAMVI) and a member of the Council of the International Society for Infectious Diseases (ISID). Since 2014, he has been recognized as a senior researcher at the Ministry of Science of Colombia. He is a professor at the Faculty of Medicine of the Fundacion Universitaria Autonoma de las Americas, in Pereira, Risaralda, Colombia, and a professor, Master in Clinical Epidemiology and Biostatistics, at Universidad Científica del Sur, Lima, Peru. He is also a non-resident adjunct faculty member at the Gilbert and Rose-Marie Chagoury School of Medicine, Lebanese American University, Beirut, Lebanon, and an external professor, Master in Research on Tropical Medicine and International Health, at Universitat de Barcelona, Spain. Additionally, an invited professor, Master in Biomedicine, at Universidad Internacional SEK, Quito, Ecuador, and a visiting professor, Master Program of Epidemiology, at Diponegoro University, Indonesia. In 2021 he was awarded the "Raul Isturiz Award" Medal of the API and, the same year, the "Jose Felix Patiño" Asclepius Staff Medal of the Colombian Medical College due to his scientific contributions to the topic of COVID-19 during the pandemic. He is currently the Editor in Chief of the journal Travel Medicine and Infectious Diseases. His Scopus H index is 55 (Google Scholar H index 77) with a total of 725 publications indexed in Scopus.

Meet the Volume Editors

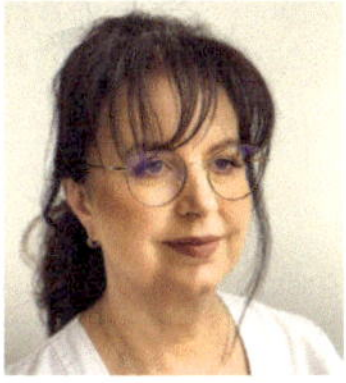

Dr. Elena Danteş is a professor at the Faculty of Medicine, "Ovidius" University of Constanta, Romania, where she is also the head of the Research and Innovation Department. With her specialization in pulmonology, Dr. Danteş has expertise in bronchology, special pulmonary function tests, somnology, and health management. Dr. Danteş is actively involved in scientific research and has participated in international grants and multicenter clinical trials, with particular emphasis on obstructive pulmonary disease, interstitial lung disease, lung cancer, and tuberculosis. She is leading the project "Establishment and Development of the South-East Regional Center for Research Career Guidance - Ad Augusta." Her accomplishments include several leadership positions (hospital medical director, department head, and county coordinator for the National Programme for Prevention, Surveillance and Control of Tuberculosis). Dr. Danteş has contributed significantly to science through her publications, including books and book chapters. In addition, her articles in prestigious databases, as well as her lectures and expert opinions, have had a lasting impact on the field of pulmonology in Romania.

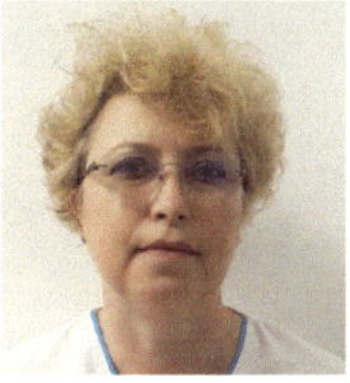

Dr. Elena Dumea is the head of Department 4 - Medical Clinical Disciplines II and a university lecturer at "Ovidius" University of Constanta, Romania. She also serves as the medical director at the Infectious Diseases Clinical Hospital Constanta. Dr. Dumea obtained her medical degree from Iasi, Romania, and completed her residency in infectious diseases and epidemiology at Constanta. Her Ph.D. research focused on HIV and viral hepatitis B co-infection, which she pursued at the University "Carol Davila," Bucharest. Dr. Dumea's research interests encompass a wide range of areas, including HIV infection, viral hepatitis, emerging infectious diseases, antibacterial activity, bacterial drug resistance, molecular microbiology, and epidemiology in relation to microbiota. She has made significant contributions to the field through the publication of numerous international research articles, books, book chapters, and congress proceedings, all centered around infectious diseases and immunocompromised hosts. Dr. Dumea's scholarly work demonstrates her dedication to advancing knowledge and understanding in the field of infectious diseases, particularly in the context of HIV, viral hepatitis, and related topics.

Contents

Preface

Histoplasmosis – A Comprehensive Study of Epidemiology, Pathogenesis, Diagnosis, and Treatment is designed to assist clinicians in effectively managing the most common cause of respiratory fungal infections, which encompass a wide spectrum of clinical manifestations from self-limiting infections to progressive, life-threatening disseminated diseases.

Histoplasmosis is a worldwide, noncontagious fungal infection caused by inhalation of fungal spores of the species *Histoplasma capsulatum*. This pathogen is widespread in certain regions with particular environmental conditions, such as areas with bird or bat droppings, organic-rich soil, and humid climates. Endemic regions of histoplasmosis include the western and southeastern parts of the United States (especially the Ohio, Mississippi, and Missouri river valleys), Central and South America, sub-Saharan Africa, eastern Asia, and Australia [1].

In this book, our authors have collaborated to provide a comprehensive overview of histoplasmosis. Chapters cover a wide range of topics, from the historical and epidemiological aspects of the disease to its clinical manifestations, diagnosis, treatment options, and preventive measures. Following the introductory section, the chapter on the epidemiology of histoplasmosis provides new insights into the changing epidemiological landscape of fungal pathogens. It also reviews the phylogenetic classification of histoplasmosis, the life cycle of infection, risk factors associated with natural habitat, modes of transmission, and hosts, and the various forms of disease manifestation in an epidemiological context. Incidence and mortality rates of histoplasmosis show high variability worldwide, are sometimes underestimated, and depend on the medical system's ability to diagnose, report, and notify cases. The following chapter presents the current epidemiologic status and knowledge gaps related to histoplasmosis on the African continent. Emphasis is placed on the lack of advanced diagnostic technologies in the context of large numbers of HIV/AIDS patients vulnerable to developing disseminated forms of the disease.

Histoplasmosis remains a significant contributor to morbidity and mortality worldwide, necessitating prevention and prophylaxis strategies, surveillance, research and development initiatives, and public health interventions [2].

Histoplasmosis presents a significant diagnostic challenge due to its nonspecific symptoms and similarity to other respiratory diseases. Chapters on clinical, imaging, and laboratory diagnosis address the common and characteristic clinical pictures, diagnostic algorithms, and bacteriological, serological, and molecular diagnostic methods. Histoplasmosis, often misdiagnosed as tuberculosis, can lead to death before it is recognized, especially in patients with HIV infection. The challenges associated with diagnosis, particularly in nonendemic areas where knowledge deficits persist, the complexity of treatment (including interactions between fungicidal drugs and cART and drug availability), and the association with other opportunistic infections (e.g., tuberculosis) have prompted specialists to devote more attention to this disease.

The chapter on HIV-associated histoplasmosis comprehensively covers all aspects of the interaction between the two conditions, as coinfection continues to pose clinical, diagnostic, and public health challenges. Since 1987, the World Health Organization (WHO) has classified histoplasmosis as an AIDS-defining disease [3].

In addition, therapeutic approaches refer to the latest advances and therapeutic strategies available to combat histoplasmosis effectively. The gold standard treatment for moderate-to-severe disseminated histoplasmosis is liposomal amphotericin B (L-AmB) [3, 4]. The liposomal formulation is preferred over the conventional deoxycholate formulation due to its lower nephrotoxicity, lower mortality rate in HIV patients, and better overall clinical success [5, 6]. Therefore, developing new drug delivery systems for treating and managing histoplasmosis is of utmost importance, especially for patients with AIDS. A chapter on treatment introduces various means of drug delivery and explores the potential of micro- and nanotechnology in the fight against histoplasmosis.

Working with experts in various fields, we have presented this complex topic concisely and efficiently, incorporating the latest research and clinical findings. Each chapter provides an in-depth examination of the topic and uses evidence-based approaches to improve the understanding and treatment of histoplasmosis.

We hope this book will serve as a valuable resource for healthcare professionals involved in diagnosing and treating histoplasmosis.

I want to express my sincere appreciation and deepest gratitude to all the authors and contributors who have given their time and expertise to the completion of this project. I hope this book will inform and inspire further advances in the understanding, prevention, and treatment of histoplasmosis.

Sincerely,

Elena Dantes
4th Department - Clinical Medical Disciplines,
Faculty of Medicine,
'Ovidius' University of Constanta,
Constanta, Romania

Clinical Hospital of Pneumophtisiology,
Constanta, Romania

Elena Dumea
4th Department - Clinical Medical Disciplines,
Faculty of Medicine,
'Ovidius' University of Constanta,
Constanta, Romania

Clinical Infectious Disease Hospital,
Constanta, Romania

References

[1] Diaz JH. Environmental and wilderness-related risk factors for histoplasmosis: more than bats in caves. Wilderness & Environmental Medicine. 2018;**29**(4):531-540. DOI: 10.1016/j.wem.2018.06.008

[2] The WHO lists multiple fungal pathogens of critical, high and medium importance for addressing with R&D, surveillance and access to diagnosis and treatment. 2022. Available from: https://gaffi.org/wp-content/uploads/WHO-FPPL-2022.pdf. [Accessed: 2023-03-03]

[3] Guidelines for diagnosing and managing disseminated histoplasmosis among people living with HIV. Washington, DC: Pan American Health Organization, and Geneva: World Health Organization; APR 2020, https://www.who.int/publications/i/item/9789240006430

[4] Azar MM, Loyd JL, Relich RF, Wheat LJ, Hage CA. Current Concepts in the Epidemiology, Diagnosis, and Management of Histoplasmosis Syndromes. Semin Respir Crit Care Med. 2020;**41**(1):13-30

[5] Arauz AB, Papineni P. Histoplasmosis. Infect Dis Clin North Am. 2021;**35**(2):471-91

[6] Johnson PC, Wheat LJ, Cloud GA, Goldman M, Lancaster D, Bamberger DM, et al. Safety and efficacy of liposomal amphotericin B compared with conventional amphotericin B for induction therapy of histoplasmosis in patients with AIDS. Ann Intern Med. 2002;**137**(2):105-9

Chapter 1

Introductory Chapter: Histoplasmosis – Challenges and New Perspectives

Elena Dantes and Elena Dumea

1. Introduction

Clinicians continue to pay attention to fungus infections because they represent a problematic pathology from various perspectives. Due to their largely non-specific symptomatology, polymorphous imaging features, and unpredictable evolution from asymptomatic disease to one that endangers life, pulmonary mycoses enter the differential diagnosis with many other disorders, whether infectious, granulomatous, neoplastic, or systemic in nature [1, 2].

A practitioner in an area with an endemic fungal illness is more equipped to facilitate a rapid and accurate diagnosis because they have a greater understanding of these diseases.

Despite being worldwide spread, histoplasmosis is better known in the Central and Midwestern parts of the United States, Ohio, and the Mississippi River Valley regions receiving the greatest attention [3]. European or African nations, however, report considerably fewer cases.

2. Challenges for histoplasmosis diagnosis

Geographic location seems to be less important today in triggering suspicion of histoplasmosis, given the extraordinary population movements (tourism, migration, or other reasons) and the numerous risk factors for host immunosuppression.

The quantity of conidia inhaled, the host's immunological status, comorbid conditions, chronic immunosuppressive medications, local access to cutting-edge research techniques, and available therapeutic choices are examples of the many additional aspects that must be considered [4].

For instance, Ocansey and colleagues pointed out in a recent article that the exact burden of this disease in African nations is unknown. The high incidence of HIV infection in the population, the sometimes-confusing diagnosis of tuberculosis, and the restricted access of the public to precise diagnostic procedures in specialized clinics all contribute to the risk of underdiagnosis of this illness. Although the rate of histoplasmosis cases has increased in the last decade and awareness among healthcare workers has improved, studies are needed on the diversity of species of the genus Histoplasma (including African species), the clinical-evolutionary features, the HIV–histoplasmosis–tuberculosis interaction, and, last but not least, the genetic predispositions of the population [5].

Histoplasmosis can be present in various ways, ranging from the localized pulmonary or cutaneous form, to affecting multiple organs in acute and chronic forms, and from self-limited to widespread. Consequently, many clinical presentations at the thoracic level, such as infiltrates, nodules, cavity lesions, and mediastinal damage, including lymphadenopathies or mediastinitis, raise the suspicion of histoplasmosis and must be distinguished from other granulomatosis like sarcoidosis, tuberculosis, or malignancy [6].

It is necessary to have an even higher suspicion of histoplasmosis (5–27%) in patients living with HIV with CD4 below 150 cells/microL [7]. The disseminated forms are predominating in the clinical presentation. The acute disseminated disease, typical in individuals with significant immunosuppression, including those living with HIV or with organ transplantation, is characterized by non-specific symptoms such as fever, sweats, fatigue, cough, dyspnea, and weight loss [8]. Additionally, extrapulmonary involvement such as hepatosplenomegaly, lymphadenopathy, injury to the skin or mucosa, digestive issues, diseases of the adrenal glands and bone marrow, or abnormalities of the central nervous system are more common [9].

The rapidity of diagnosis depends on the sensitivity and specificity of the laboratory instruments used in conjunction with the time after exposure, the organ affected, the acute or chronic course, and the extent of infection (localized or disseminated). A rapid diagnosis can be made by enzyme immunoassay (EIA) to detect histoplasma antigens in bronchioloalveolar lavage fluid, urine, blood, or cerebrospinal fluid (CSF).

In acute diffuse pulmonary forms, serologic and antigen tests have high sensitivity several weeks after exposure. In localized mediastinal, adenophatic, or pulmonary forms (nodules), these tests may be negative or have lower sensitivity. To confirm the diagnosis, the physician must request staining of tissues for fungi in combination with culture from blood, sputum, or other tissues (adenophatic, lung masses, or bone marrow) [9]. Microscopic detection of yeasts in clinical specimens and growth of molds in cultures are the gold standards for confirming the diagnosis.

Differential diagnosis can be challenging, especially with other granulomatosis, such as sarcoidosis. Therefore, histoplasmosis should be ruled out in patients with mediastinal lymphadenopathy, nodules, infiltrative lesions, and even elevated angiotensin-converting enzyme serum levels if histopathologic examination revealed a noncaseating granuloma before initiating immunosuppressive treatment for sarcoidosis.

Several conditions must be met to support the diagnosis of histoplasmosis. First, the physician should think of this pathology when the symptoms and radiological manifestations (focal or diffuse airspace disease, lymphadenopathy, cavitary upper lobes, thick-walled bullae, and fibrotic mediastinitis) are compatible, especially in cases of high local endemicity [1, 3, 4]. Secondly, access to a wide range of tests that suggest and confirm histoplasmosis is desirable. Identifying *Histoplasma capsulatum* in culture from biopsy specimens, sputum, or bronchoalveolar lavage supports a precise positive diagnosis.

3. New perspectives for the treatment of histoplasmosis

The decision to initiate treatment for histoplasmosis depends on the form and clinical presentation of the disease: Self-limited forms usually do not require treatment, in contrast to moderate and severe forms with persistent symptoms, extensive lesions, or chronic conditions. In these cases, administering an effective treatment with minimal side effects, such as lipid amphotericin B followed by itraconazole for a sufficient period of time, is reasonable [10].

The use of nanocarriers for drug delivery has demonstrated their potential as an alternative and versatile technological platform for the treatment of intracellular infections caused by fungi of the species *H. capsulatum* [11]. However, future research is needed to improve the outcomes of this disease.

The chapters included in this book address all of these challenges related to the epidemiology, diagnosis, and treatment of histoplasmosis.

Author details

Elena Dantes[1,2*] and Elena Dumea[1,3]

1 4th Department - Clinical Medical Disciplines, Faculty of Medicine, 'Ovidius' University of Constanta, Constanta, Romania

2 Clinical Hospital of Pneumophtisiology, Constanta, Romania

3 Clinical Infectious Disease Hospital, Constanta, Romania

*Address all correspondence to: elena.dantes@gmail.com

References

[1] Ekeng BE, Davies AA, Osaigbovo II, Warris A, Oladele RO, Denning DW. Pulmonary and extrapulmonary manifestations of fungal infections misdiagnosed as tuberculosis: The need for prompt diagnosis and management. Journal of Fungi. 2022;**8**(5):460. DOI: 10.3390/jof8050460

[2] Shah KK, Pritt BS, Alexander MP. Histopathologic review of granulomatous inflammation. Journal of Clinical Tuberculosis and Other Mycobacterial Diseases. 2017;**7**:1-12. DOI: 10.1016/j.jctube.2017.02.001

[3] Azar MM, Loyd JL, Relich RF, Wheat LJ, Hage CA. Current concepts in the epidemiology, diagnosis, and management of histoplasmosis syndromes. Seminars in Respiratory and Critical Care Medicine. 2020;**41**(1):13-30. DOI: 10.1055/s-0039-1698429. Epub 2020 Jan 30

[4] Kauffman CA. Histoplasmosis: A clinical and laboratory update. Clinical Microbiology Reviews. Jan 2007;**20**(1):115-132. DOI: 10.1128/CMR.00027-06

[5] Ocansey BK, Kosmidis C, Agyei M, Dorkenoo AM, Ayanlowo OO, Oladele RO, et al. Histoplasmosis in Africa: Current perspectives, knowledge gaps, and research priorities. PLoS Neglected Tropical Diseases. 2022;**16**(2):e0010111. DOI: 10.1371/journal.pntd.0010111

[6] Wheat LJ, Conces D, Allen SD, et al. Pulmonary histoplasmosis syndromes: Recognition, diagnosis, and management. Seminars in Respiratory and Critical Care Medicine. 2004;**25**:129

[7] Myint T, Leedy N, Villacorta Cari E, Wheat LJ. HIV-associated histoplasmosis: Current perspectives. HIV AIDS (Auckl). 2020;**12**:113-125. DOI: 10.2147/HIV.S185631

[8] Saullo JL, Miller RA. Updates on histoplasmosis in solid organ transplantation. Current Fungal Infection Reports. 2022;**16**(4):165-178. DOI: 10.1007/s12281-022-00441-1. Epub 2022 Sep 8

[9] Couppié P, Herceg K, Bourne-Watrin M, Thomas V, Blanchet D, Alsibai KD, et al. The broad clinical spectrum of disseminated histoplasmosis in HIV-infected patients: A 30 years' experience in French Guiana. Journal of Fungi. 2019;**5**(4):115. DOI: 10.3390/jof5040115

[10] Wheat J, Sarosi G, McKinsey D, Hamill R, Bradsher R, Johnson P, et al. Practice guidelines for the management of patients with histoplasmosis. Clinical Infectious Diseases. 2000;**30**(4):688-695. DOI: 10.1086/313752

[11] Mejia SP, Sanchez A, Vasquez V, Orozco J. Functional nanocarriers for delivering itraconazole against fungal intracellular infections. Frontiers in Pharmacology. 2021;**12**:685391

Chapter 2

Epidemiology of Histoplasmosis

Nela Daniela Efrim, Elena Dumea and Roxana Carmen Cernat

Abstract

More prevalent than initially considered, histoplasmosis is primarily a non-contagious disease of the reticuloendothelial system, producing a broad spectrum of clinical manifestations, ranging from asymptomatic or self-limited infection, in immunocompetent patients to life-threatening, disseminated disease in immunocompromised ones. The causative agent is *H. capsulatum*, a thermally dimorphic, intracellular fungus, discovered in 1906, by the pathologist Samuel Darling, when examined tissues from a young man whose death was mistakenly attributed to miliary tuberculosis. Since then, histoplasmosis was described on six continents, with high and low endemicity areas. *H. capsulatum* is a soil-based fungus, commonly associated with river valleys in the temperate zone, and with the presence of bird and bat guano. Infection occurs when saprophytic spores are inhaled and change to the pathogenic yeast in the lungs, where *H. capsulatum* overcomes many obstacles to cause host injuries. Depending on geographic distribution, morphology, and clinical symptoms, three varieties have been historically recognized, two of them (*var. capsulatum* and *var. duboisii*) being pathogen to humans, and the third (*var. farciminosum*) has predominantly been described as an equine pathogen. In endemic areas, patients with AIDS or people who receive immunosuppressive therapies should be counseled to avoid high-risk activities; otherwise, precautionary measures should be taken.

Keywords: widely distributed, changing epidemiology, cellular immunity, occupational disease, global burden

1. Introduction

Fungi represent the second largest estimated species numbers after insects. Their kingdom comprises a huge variety of microorganisms, the newer estimates, based on data acquired from molecular methods, have predicted from 1.5 million fungal species, in some conservative estimates [1–4], to a spectacular 13.2 million, in others [5, 6], less than 150.000 species being merely cataloged to date [5–8]. For many years, it was believed that fungi were clinically insignificant, but the increased incidence of invasive fungal infections during the past 20 years has contradicted this hypothesis [9].

Compared to the enormous biomass of fungal species, the number of human pathogenic fungi is minuscule, but they exert a profound, global impact on human health. Billions of people are infected, [10] fungi causing more than a billion skin infections, more than 100 million mucosal infections, 10 million serious allergies [11], and more than 1.5 million deaths every year [4, 12]. Worldwide, mortality due to fungal infections exceeds that from breast cancer and malaria and is comparable to that owing to tuberculosis and HIV, exerting a major threat to human health and, consequently, a huge burden to global healthcare budgets [11, 12].

In the past 15 years, in the world landscape, new species of fungi were yearly discovered at a rate varying from 2100 to 2600 species, most of them in Asia (41%) and Europe (23%), and a small part even in Antarctica (0.5%) (**Figure 1**) [8].

Also, the number of clinically relevant fungal species continued to grow, this fact being clearly demonstrated by their increasing number in the Atlas of Clinical Fungi, of which the first edition, in 1995, contained 320 species, while the fourth edition of the same book, published in 2020, counts more than 660 fungal species [13, 14].

Climate change will have an impact on the way we interact with our environment and, because fungi can easily adapt to these changes, the overall epidemiological picture of pathogens will also modify. This will likely expose us to varieties of fungi that humans and animals have never interacted with. Due to climate change, the diversity and number of soil microorganisms will undoubtedly change, as already seen with endemic fungi (**Figure 2**) and with the emergence of new fungal pathogens [4].

Furthermore, modern life-saving medical procedures and aggressive medical treatments may affect normal immune functions and, paradoxically, have given rise to large groups of people at risk for fungal infections. Patients at high risk include those with AIDS, those receiving immunosuppressive therapy, transplant recipients, and certain surgeries and those in intensive care settings [15, 16].

There is a growing body of evidence supporting the concern that climate change will affect the morbidity and mortality rates of infectious diseases, and that fungi will play an increasing role as primary or secondary pathogens [4].

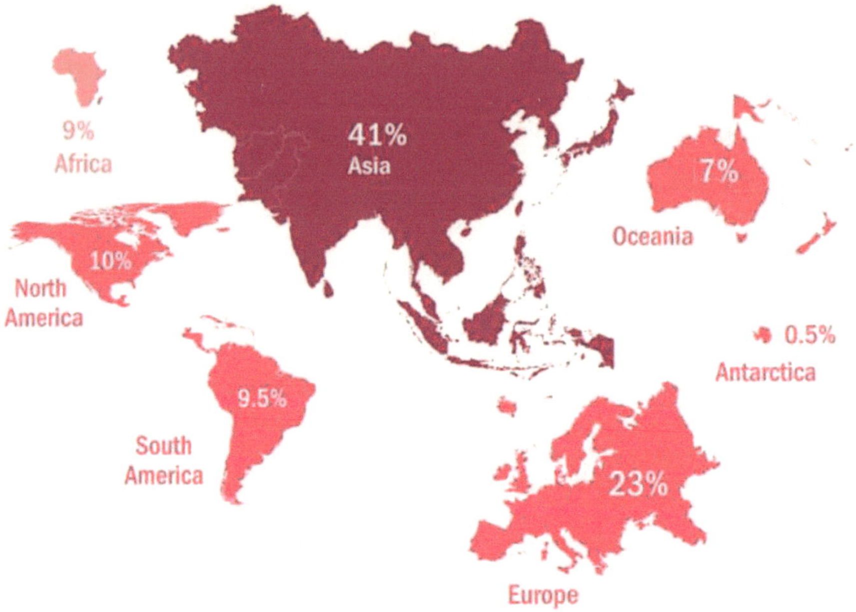

Figure 1.
Graphic map of the world's continents showing the uneven distribution of newly described species of fungi. The size of each continent is proportional to the global percentage of new species published from there and mainly reflects both the quantity of taxonomic expertise and the presence of undescribed species in those areas. Also, the map reflects the location of most research activity and taxonomic expertise. Artwork Creative Services/ RBG Kew. [8]. https://nph.onlinelibrary.wiley.com/doi/10.1002/ppp3.10148.

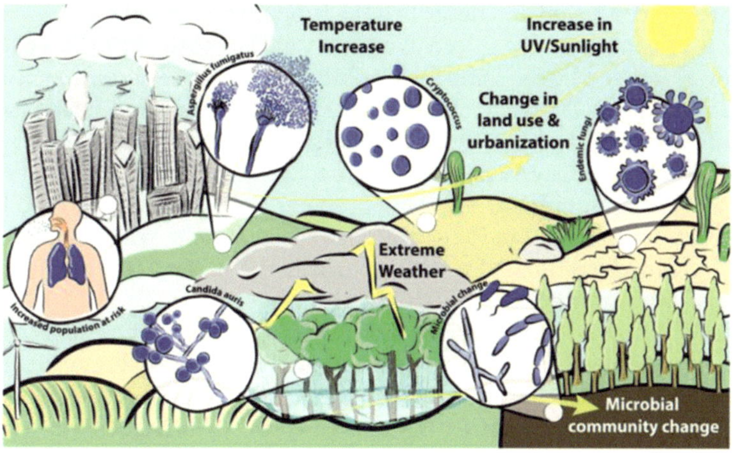

Figure 2.
Schematic overview of changes in the epidemiological landscape of fungal pathogens and associated changes in environmental parameters [4]. https://www.mdpi.com/2309-608X/7/5/367.

To infect and cause disease in healthy humans, true pathogenic fungi should meet four basic criteria: (i) growth at elevated human body temperatures, (ii) bypassing around or penetrating through surface host barriers, (iii) secretion of lytic enzymes for acquiring nutrients from the host tissues, and (iv) evasion or resistance to the host's immune defense systems. The fungi that infect previous healthy humans represent a small group, many more invasive fungal infections now occurring in patients with underlying serious illnesses [15, 17].

The severity and outcome of infection is determined by both the extent of the exposure to the organism and by the immune status of the patient [18].

Therefore, with the expansion of the susceptible population and the increase in the frequency of mycotic infections, the mortality due to invasive mycoses was estimated at one and a half million deaths annually [12, 18].

Histoplasmosis is the most prevalent cause of fungal respiratory infections and has a vast spectrum of clinical manifestations, ranging from a self-limited, acute, influenza-like illness to a progressive disseminated life-threatening infection [19, 20].

2. Historical milestones for *H. capsulatum* and histoplasmosis

The first description of the disease was made in December 1905 by the pathologist Samuel Taylor Darling, when examining smears of tissues and bone marrow from a young carpenter from Martinique, whose death was mistakenly attributed to acute miliary tuberculosis. Darling found an enormous number of small, oval, and round bodies, located in alveolar epithelial cells and in the plasma of the spleen and rib marrow, which he attributed to a parasite resembling to be closely related to Leishmania. He proposed the name *H. capsulatum*, because of the similarity of its halo with a capsule [21].

Only a few years later, in 1912, Henrique da Rocha Lima, inferring the mycotic nature of this pathogen, offered a correct depiction of the microorganism and recognized *H. capsulatum* as a fungus [22].

The first case diagnosed in humans with an acute disseminated form of histoplasmosis was that of a 6-year-old child who died in 1932 [23].

De Monbreun cultivated and described the fungus from blood cultures taken 2 days before death and from the spleen at autopsy, in 1934. Also, in 1939, a culture of *H. capsulatum* was isolated by the same De Monbreun from a case occurring in a dog. He noticed that primary isolated colonies contained both mycelial and yeast phases from the fungus and was able to convert the mycelial phase to the yeast-like one by inoculating susceptible animals. Ciferri and Radaelli managed to convert a strain of *H. capsulatum* to the yeast form by cultural methods, growing it on blood agar at 37°C [22].

In 1941, Zarafonetis and Lindberg prepared histoplasmin, which is a filtrate of a culture of *H. capsulatum*, in the mycelial phase [24]. On the African continent, histoplasmosis was first reported in 1942 by Duncan [25].

Four decades after it was first described, histoplasmosis was considered a rare, acute, and lethal disease, based on reported cases in the medical literature. Starting with 1945, this belief was contradicted by several investigators, arguing that, in fact, fatal cases were the exception rather than the rule, the infection occurring in certain areas of the USA, in an asymptomatic or benign form, rarely recognized clinically by physicians and being misdiagnosed as tuberculosis [26].

In 1945, Christie and Peterson were the first using histoplasmin in an epidemiological survey, which clearly demonstrated the correlation between pulmonary calcifications and histoplasmin sensitivity in tuberculin-negative persons [27].

Also in 1945, Palmer confirmed the existence of subclinical cases of histoplasmosis, which reacted positively to the histoplasmin skin test [28]. Only 1 year later, the same Palmer demonstrated that the highest frequency of histoplasmin reactors was discovered in the same area of the USA, where clinical cases of histoplasmosis had been repeatedly diagnosed [28].

Furcolow demonstrated in 1949 the development of asymptomatic, benign, pulmonary infiltrations, indistinguishable from tuberculosis, in a group of tuberculin-negative, histoplasmin-positive persons, using a series of chest radiographs over a three-year period [29].

In 1949, Emmons isolated macroconidia of *H. capsulatum* from soil samples, by examining saline suspension by direct microscopy and demonstrated that the fungus goes through a developmental saprophytic cycle in soil [30].

A first description as a new variant of Histoplasma was made by Vanbreuseghem in 1952, and, in honor of Professor Albert Dubois, who provided the isolates, the fungus was named *H. capsulatum* var. duboisii [31].

In 1969, Edwards and colleagues published the first map of histoplasmin skin reactivity in the USA, illustrating the endemicity of the disease primarily in the Ohio and Mississippi River valleys [32].

Kwon-Chung, in 1972, reported the observation of sexual reproduction of *H. capsulatum* [33] and, only a few months later, he stated that Emmonsiella capsulata is the teleomorph or sexual stage, resulting from the sexual compatibility + and – mating types of *H. capsulatum* (asexual stage or anamorph) [34].

In 2003, Hwang and his colleagues conducted the first large genomic study, which identified and compared genes that exhibit phase-specific patterns of expression in *H. capsulatum*, providing a more complete description of both the yeast and mycelial phases of the fungus [35].

Using the multilocus sequence typing (MLST) method, in 2003, Kasuga performed the first analysis across the global distribution of the Histoplasma species. He found intermixed isolates from the three variants of Histoplasma in multiple phylogenetic clades and refined the classification of the fungus by identifying eight phylogenetic clades of *H. capsulatum* [36].

In 2014, it was documented and reported transplacental transmission of *H. capsulatum* in a series of patients [37].

For the first time in the medical literature, cases of mixed infection with different mating types of Histoplasma were described in two patients living with HIV in 2019, in an endemic area of Brazil [38].

In 2022, *H. capsulatum* was first detected by molecular techniques in the soil and penguin excreta collected from the Antarctic Peninsula [39].

To guide research, development, and more robust public health actions, in October 2022 WHO developed the first fungal priority pathogens list (WHO FPPL) which included Histoplasma spp. in the high-priority group [40].

3. The epidemiologic triad of histoplasmosis

Like other infectious diseases, histoplasmosis results from the complex interaction between the pathogen and the susceptible host in a favorable environment that supports the transmission of the agent from the source to that host.

3.1 Agent

Histoplasmosis is a worldwide distributed non-contagious fungal infection caused by *H. capsulatum*.

3.1.1 Characteristics of H. capsulatum

H. capsulatum is a thermally dimorphic, primary systemic, and endemic fungal pathogen. *Thermal dimorphism* implies the existence of the pathogen in two different forms, depending on the temperatures. *H. capsulatum* presents itself, either in a hyaline mold in the environment or in the laboratory at 25–35°C, or in an intracellular budding yeast form in mammalian tissues or when grown on enriched medium in the laboratory at 37°C [41]. Thermal dimorphism is not restricted to the fungus morphology, but also implies the shift between the saprophytic, avirulent mycelial form, and the parasitic, pathogenic yeast form [42].

The fungus is characterized as a *primary pathogen* because of its ability to cause infection both in previous healthy individuals and immunocompromised hosts and *systemic* for its tendency to involve deep viscera after dissemination from the lungs [17, 41].

In 95% of immunocompetent individuals, the infection with *H. capsulatum* evolves usually benign and asymptomatic. Histoplasmosis is life-threatening particularly in immunocompromised patients, clinical manifestations, and the prognosis of the disease depending on the size inoculum and virulence of the infecting strain [17]. Since the beginning of HIV pandemic in 1980s, histoplasmosis has also been considered an AIDS-defining illness starting with 1987 [43–45].

H. capsulatum is also known as an *endemic* fungus, its natural habitat being delimitated to specific geographic regions and infection is acquired by inhalation of the spores from that specific environment or geographic area. Endemic areas for histoplasmosis include Mid-western and South-eastern parts of the United States (especially Ohio, Mississippi, and Missouri river valleys), Central and South America, sub-Saharan Africa, Eastern Asia, and Australia [46].

In the kingdom of fungi, *H. capsulatum* specie belongs to the phylum Ascomycota, family Onygenaceae [47, 48].

In fact, *H. capsulatum* is the asexual (anamorph) state of the fungus, which has a heterothallic form, designated Ajellomyces capsulatus or Emmonsiella capsulata (teleomorph or sexual state). The last is the perfect state of the fungus, being capable of producing sexual spores. When encountered and combined onto a sporulating medium, mating types (+) and (−) produce fruiting bodies containing asci. Although the mating type ratio in soil is 1:1, in isolates from patients the (−) mating type is found two to seven times more frequently than the opposite mating type [34, 49–52].

3.1.2 Classifications and mycology of H. capsulatum

H. capsulatum was historically classified, according to geographic distribution, morphology, host-association, and clinical manifestations, into three varieties: (i) *H. capsulatum var. capsulatum*, responsible for classic histoplasmosis, causing pulmonary and disseminated infection worldwide; (ii) *H. capsulatum var. duboisii*, causing predominantly skin and bone lesions, mostly in the African continent; and (iii) *H. capsulatum var. farciminosum*, predominantly responsible for epizootic lymphangitis in equines. Morphologically, the two variants of *H. capsulatum* pathogenic for humans, cultured at 25°C, are macroscopically and microscopically indistinguishable. Growth is obtained on blood agar, chocolate agar, or Sabouraud's agar. Macroscopically, the mold is slowly growing as white (A type) or tan to brown (B type) colonies, usually in 2 to 6 weeks. The A type grows faster, is nonpigmented, and loses its ability to produce spores when subcultured. Also, yeast cells produced from the A type are less virulent in mice than those obtained from B type [49]. Microscopic evaluation of the mold reveals the mycelium, with septate, hyaline hyphae producing two types of conidia (**Figure 3**). Macroconidia are large (8–15 μm in diameter), spherical, thick-walled bodies formed on short, hyaline conidiospores. Their surface is decorated with spike-like or finger-like projections, hence the name tuberculate macroconidia, which represents the typical microscopic structure for presumptive diagnostic. Microconidia are small (2–4 μm in diameter), smooth-walled, oval to pyriform bodies, sessile or attached on short stalks, at right angles, on the sides of the hyphae. These conidia are considered infectious forms due to the small size that allows them to penetrate up to the level of the alveoli.

When cultured at 37°C on enriched media (such BHIA—brain heart infusion agar containing blood), both *H. capsulatum* var. capsulatum and *H. capsulatum* var. duboisii develop smooth, creamy, moist, and yeast-like colonies. Initially, the colony

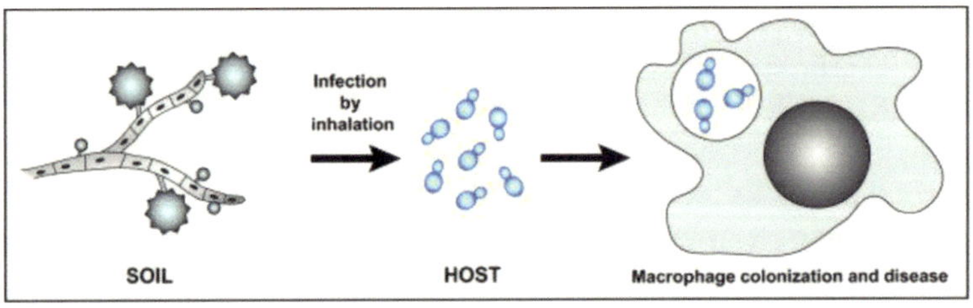

Figure 3.
H. capsulatum grows in the soil as a saprophytic mold (left). After inhalation, triggered by the temperature of the mammalian host, converts to the pathogenic yeast form (center) capable of intracellular replication within host macrophages (right) [53]. https://bmcmicrobiol.biomedcentral.com/articles/10.1186/1471-2180-11-216.

appears white or cream-colored and becomes gray with age. Microscopically, there are differences in yeast-like colonies between the two varieties of Histoplasma. Numerous round to oval budding, uninucleate yeast-like cells are revealed, small (2–4 μm) and thin-walled for *H. capsulatum* var. capsulatum, and large (8–15 μm) and thick-walled for *H. capsulatum* var. duboisii. The yeast cell reproduces by polar budding, resulting in the characteristic narrow bridge appearance (**Figure 3**) between the mother cell and the daughter cell [48, 49, 54].

The cultures of *H. capsulatum* are associated with high individual risk and require Class II Biological Safety (BSCII) precautions [49].

Between 1986 and 1992, Vincent, Spitzer, Keath, and their colleagues performed genetic studies by comparing soil, human or veterinary isolates and finally classified *H. capsulatum* into six genotypes or classes, correlated with a peculiar geographic distribution [55–57].

Using DNA sequence variations of protein-coding genes of isolates from six continents, in 2003, Kasuga and colleagues defined eight phylogenetic clades grouped in seven phylogenetic species, as follows: (i) North American class 1 clade (NAm 1); (ii) North American class 2 clade (NAm 2); (iii) Latin American group A clade (LAm A); (iv) Latin American group B clade (LAm B); (v) Australian clade; (vi) Netherlands (Indonesian?) clade; (vii) Eurasian clade—harboring isolates from China, India, Thailand, Egypt, and England; (viii) African clade. Each clade represents a genetically isolated specie, with only one exception, the Eurasian clade, which originated from LAm A specie. Thus, the original classification of Histoplasma became obsolete, *H. capsulatum* var. capsulatum being found in all phylogenetic species, *H. capsulatum* var. duboisii belonging to African phylogenetic species, and *H. capsulatum* var. farciminosum being placed in NAm 2 and African phylogenetic species and, mainly, in the Eurasian clade [36].

The studies carried out by Teixeira and colleagues refined this classification, and the number of phylogenetic species was increased to 11. He split LAm A and LAm B phylogenetic species into LAm A1 and LAm A2, respectively LAm B1 and LAm B2. Also, he added to the classification two new phylogenetic species, Rio de Janeiro—RJ, and a bat-associated clade—BAC1 (from Mexico), the last one being renamed NAm 3 for his similarities with NAm 2 [58].

In 2019, another improvement in phylogenetic classification of histoplasma was made due to Damasceno's et al. research on HIV-positive patient isolates from the northeastern part of Brazil. Two new monophyletic species were added to the previous classification of *H. capsulatum*, named Northeast BR 1 and Northeast BR 2 [45].

Using whole-genome data, Sepúlveda advanced a more robust analysis, dividing 30 isolates into 5 independently evolving lineages, which he considered separate phylogenetic species. He proposed another classification of the genus Histoplasma as follows: *H. capsulatum* sensu stricto (referring to the Panamanian lineage—H81), *H. mississippiense* (formerly known as NAm 1), *H. ohiense* (formerly known as NAm 2), *H. suramericanum* (formerly known as LAm A), and African clade [59].

Depending on the chemical differences of the wall, the yeast form of *H. capsulatum* is classified as chemotype I, when the α-(1,3)-glucan layer is absent and the fibers are entirely β-linked or chemotype II, when the wall contains a mixture of an α and β-(1,3)-glucans [60].

Chemotype I appears to be more virulent, being accountable for most infections in immunocompetent individuals in North America. Additionally, in mouse models, same chemotype causes more severe forms of disease than chemotype II [61].

3.1.3 Life cycle of H. capsulatum

The life cycle of the fungus does not necessarily require the yeast-phase transition and infection of a mammalian host. Rather, human infections are believed to be accidental, the resulting systemic mycoses being an unfortunate consequence of the fungus ability to adapt during its evolution as a species when encounter the hostile environment of the human body [61–63].

In the soil, the mold form of *H. capsulatum* may reproduce by either sexual or asexual process. In sexual reproduction, the haploid nuclei of two opposite mating types, if encountered, fuse to form a diploid nucleus, which then divides by meiosis and produces ascospores. The mycelia are also able to asexually reproduce by mitotic division, the process being known as conidiation. As a result of conidiation is the production of vegetative budding spores: macroconidia and microconidia. These conidia can germinate in the soil and further, depending on temperature, can adopt either the mold or the yeast form [64]. When the soil is disrupted, conidia and fragments of hyphal mycelia become aerosolized and are inhaled by a susceptible host. Once entered the lungs of the host, triggered by the warmer body temperature, these infectious propagules germinate within distal bronchioles and pulmonary alveoli and convert to budding yeast. The yeast is phagocytized by immune cells and reaches the regional lymph nodes, from where it can spread to other parts of the body through the bloodstream (**Figure 4**) [48, 62, 64].

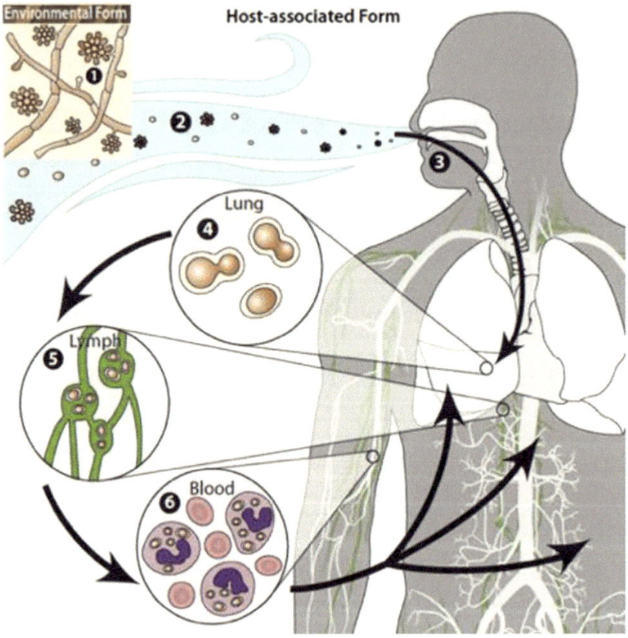

Figure 4.
Life cycle of H. capsulatum. The environmental form of H. capsulatum is a mold (1) with aerial hyphae, producing saprophytic spores (2) which are aerosolized and inhaled by the susceptible host (3). In the lungs (4), their transformation into the parasitic form of yeast takes place and, consequently, their dissemination through the lymphatic system (5) and then through the blood (6) to other organs. https://www.cdc.gov/fungal/diseases/histoplasmosis/causes.html

3.2 Host

The incubation period of the disease is not known with certainty [65], but some authors suggest an interval between 3 to 21 days [46, 66].

The extent and severity of the clinical picture of the disease are determined by the amount of conidia inhaled, the effectiveness of the host's cell-mediated immunity and the virulence of the infective strain of Histoplasma [48, 62, 67].

In most immunocompetent individuals, the infection is mildly symptomatic or even asymptomatic. About 95–99% of the primary infections in endemic areas have never been diagnosed as being histoplasmosis. However, acute severe pneumonia and chronic progressive pulmonary histoplasmosis can also occur in a healthy person if many conidia are inhaled. In individuals with impaired cell-mediated immunity, even a small inoculum or a previously considered avirulent strain can cause life-threatening to fatal disease [41, 48, 54, 62, 67, 68]. *H. capsulatum* primary infection can remain in a latent, quiescent state, without any symptoms, even for decades, and can reactivate if the host's immunosuppression occurs [48, 49, 68].

Patients at high risk for reactivating latent infection and developing disseminated histoplasmosis are those chronically receiving corticosteroids or chemotherapy, those receiving anti-cytokine therapies (tumor necrosis factor alpha or gamma interferons antagonists), individuals who have received solid organ transplantation, and patients with advanced HIV infection [63, 67]. Additional risk factors for histoplasmosis include smoking [69], COPD [70], extreme ages (infants younger than 2 years old, elderly older than 50 years old) [71], and genetics deficiencies (IFN-γ receptor 1 deficiency or histocompatibility complex haplotypes) [72, 73].

Histoplasmosis is reported among wild animals (rodents, marsupials, sloths, spotted skunks, opossums, baboons) and domestic animals such as cats, dogs, and horses [52, 65].

Some animal reservoirs could be used as sentinels in epidemiological surveillance of the disease in a defined territory, due to potentially wider environmental exposures and limited travel [74].

3.3 Environment

3.3.1 Natural habitat

The existence of *H. capsulatum* has been reported on all continents, including recently in Antarctica [39].

Although, in the past, histoplasmosis was reported in tropical and subtropical areas between latitudes 45°N and 35°S, autochthonous cases have been reported, in recent decades, in both Canada and Patagonia, demonstrating a geographical dispersion at extreme latitudes of *H. capsulatum*. The wide geographic spread of the fungus may be the result of behavioral changes in its natural reservoirs and dispersers as well as climatic changes in its natural habitat [75].

The natural habitat for *H. capsulatum* is soil enriched with bat guano or bird droppings, which favors the growth of its mycelial phase. Once contaminated, the fungus persists for many years in the soil under black bird roosts and chicken farms, even after the birds no longer stay in the area [15, 49]. Numerous other species of birds were strongly associated with *H. capsulatum* habitats: grackles, pigeons, starlings, and oil birds [76].

The fungus prefers the dark areas where temperatures are 22–29°C, near watercourses with humidity above 60%, and with porous, slightly acidic soil, high in nitrogen, and phosphorus elements [45, 68]. These conditions allow this geophilic-saprotrophic fungus to absorb the required nutrients from organic matter in soil and to unimpeded proliferate in the environment [47, 62]. Conidia of *H. capsulatum* were also isolated from air and water specimens [76].

3.3.2 Transmission routes

Typically, the portal of entry of *H. capsulatum* is the lung and the main transmission mode is indirect, through the inhalation of airborne infectious propagules from the environment. However, few cases of histoplasmosis have been attributed to indoor transmission of Histoplasma spores through building air handling systems or cleaning air ducts [77], through inhaling contaminated cocaine [78] and aerosolized conidia produced by composed organic fertilizers [79].

The infection is not contagious, airborne transmission by nasal secretions or direct host-to-host transmission of the fungus have never been established [61, 64, 75, 80]. Although exceptional, the vertical transmission route has been reported in newborns of mothers who manifested the disease in the last trimester of pregnancy, while receiving anti-TNF therapy or in the setting of HIV infection [80].

Also, donor-to-recipient fungal transmission through an infected allograft has been clearly documented [81, 82]. The incidence is rare (1 case per 1000 person-years) most infections occurring within 1–2 years after transplantation [83].

The transcutaneous route of transmission has also been suggested, especially in *H. capsulatum* var. duboisii, but the evidence is sparse, supported in some studies by the appearance of lesions at acupuncture needle pricks after mud baths and tattoos [65, 67, 84], or by sharing needles with an infected patient [85].

3.3.3 Risk factors for epidemiological process

Bats play a more important role than terrestrial mammal hosts in dispersion and transmission of the infection because of their ability to cross long distances and to spread the mycelia. The infected bats are also natural reservoirs of *H. capsulatum*, returning the fungus to the environment through their urine, feces, and carcasses. Although immune to disease, starlings and black birds contribute to the spreading of spores on their feathers, beaks, claws, and feet over short distances and, on the other hand, favor the mycelial growth in the soil through their droppings rich in nitrogen and phosphorus [48, 49, 75]. Wind, storms, airstreams in bat caves, and other natural environmental phenomenon are promoting factors for the epidemiological process. Poorly protected water supply basins or wells can be contaminated by water from sanitary and storm sewers that have washed away the soil, manure, dust, and decayed wood harboring *H. capsulatum* [86].

Studies performed to investigate the longevity of *H. capsulatum* in composed organic fertilizers obtained from hens and chicken manure demonstrated that some of them are associated with an important risk of infection by fungal-aerosolized conidia [75, 79].

Invasion and deforestation of the natural habitats of bats and birds and accelerated urbanization by disrupting the environment by excavation and construction are significant risk factors for producing air-borne conidiospores of *H. capsulatum*, and consequently infections [46, 75]. Once predominant in rural areas, histoplasmosis became more prevalent in urban areas and was classified as an occupational and recreational disease. Builders, constructors, housekeepers, farmers, gardeners, tree cutters, hunters, speleologists, archeologists, and microbiology laboratory workers are at increased risk of acquiring occupational histoplasmosis. Outdoor recreational activities such as traveling in endemic areas, cave exploration, bird and bat watching, golf and tennis courses, and visiting amusement parks could be at risk of acquiring the fungus [45, 66, 79].

Histoplasmosis appears to affect all age groups from 13 months to 70 years [65], with a predominance of cases in men (2:1 male-to-female ratio), which might be related to outdoor occupational exposure [87].

3.3.4 Forms of manifestation of the epidemiological process

An "*endemic* disease" is, by definition, one "occurring frequently in a particular region or population." Histoplasmosis occurs, with low or greater endemicity, in some known areas, more frequently in some populations (e.g., up to 25% of people living with HIV in hyper-endemic areas develop manifest histoplasmosis) [88]. In certain locations from Americas, and parts of Asia and of Africa, skintest surveys indicate that more than half of the population acquired histoplasmosis early in life [89].

The *epidemic* form of histoplasmosis is usually associated with outbreaks. An outbreak is defined as involving at least two cases, usually originating from the same known source [77].

Outbreaks of histoplasmosis are closely related to exposure, especially of immunocompetent individuals, to a large amount of aerosolized conidia of *H. capsulatum* during occupational activities that disturb vegetation and soil, containing bird or bat droppings, or during recreational trips to abandoned archeological sites or bat caves [45, 90, 91]. Although most infections are not outbreak-associated [91], individuals acquiring histoplasmosis during an outbreak may experience more intense exposures and thus potentially develop more severe disease than persons sporadically infected [90]. Due to high dose exposure during outbreaks, attack rates have been estimated at 50–100% [92].

During outbreaks and in high-risk groups, the incidence of cases is higher than 100 per 100,000 inhabitants [52]. The epidemic form of manifestation of the epidemiological process is mainly described in some Latin American countries, but numerous reports also described outbreaks of histoplasmosis in the US and Canada prior to the 1980s [77]. In recent years, this type of exposure affects more people due to the shift of outbreaks from rural to urban areas [4].

Sporadic or isolated cases are related to passive exposure during normal daily activities, are usually diagnosed outside areas recognized as endemic, and cannot be associated with a specific situation or known source of infection [48, 74]. Estimative data suggest that only 1% of sporadic infections are symptomatic [92].

Histoplasmosis occurs infrequently in persons living in non-endemic areas, but increasingly imported cases are recognized and diagnosed in immigrants or after traveling in endemic locations, especially in individuals with impaired cellular immunity [89].

3.3.5 Distribution and burden of the disease

Histoplasmosis has a wide distribution around the globe, being reported on all continents excepting Antarctica.

The real burden of the disease seems to be underestimated because it is frequently misdiagnosed as tuberculosis [52], community-acquired pneumonia or other acute lower respiratory tract infections [93], and underdiagnosed due to poor availability of diagnostic tests [94]. In addition, the incidence of the disease is poorly described even in areas known to be endemic, since histoplasmosis is not a nationally notifiable condition by the clinicians, even in the USA [93]. However, recent global estimates found almost 500,000 cases of histoplasmosis and approximately 100,000 cases of disseminated histoplasmosis occurring annually [12].

Although exposure to *H. capsulatum* was initially thought to be limited to the traditional area described by the well-known Edwards' map, with the onset of the HIV pandemic in 1980s and the emergence of new cases outside this area, this theory has been challenged [69].

Consequently, an increasing number of reported cases, both from areas previously known and from areas not known to be endemic, disclosed a wider geographic distribution of the fungus than historically described (**Figure 5**) [69, 94].

According to Global Action for Fungal Infections (Gaffi), the case fatality rate of disseminated histoplasmosis is 15–30%, if timely treated, and more than 80,000 deaths with this diagnostic were estimated annually [95].

Since 1987, the disseminated form of histoplasmosis is considered an AIDS-defining event [96]. In people living with HIV (PLHIV) in endemic areas, the annual incidence of progressive disseminated histoplasmosis (PDH) is about 5%, with mortality rates remaining high, even with the availability of antiretroviral therapy (ART) [97].

In hyper-endemic areas up to 25% of PLHIV develop clinical histoplasmosis [88] and an estimated 20% will develop PDH, with fatal prognosis without timely diagnostic and therapy [97]. The annual incidence of the disease was estimated from 0.1 to 100 cases per 100,000 inhabitants, with the lowest rates described in temperate territories and the highest in tropical areas [52]. The incidence varies within continents and territories, histoplasmosis being known to be highly endemic in central and eastern areas of North America (in the Ohio and Mississippi River Valleys), Central and South America, and parts of sub-Saharan Africa [46, 62, 63]. The disease is also endemic in patchy regions of Southeast Asia and Australia [98, 99] and sporadically

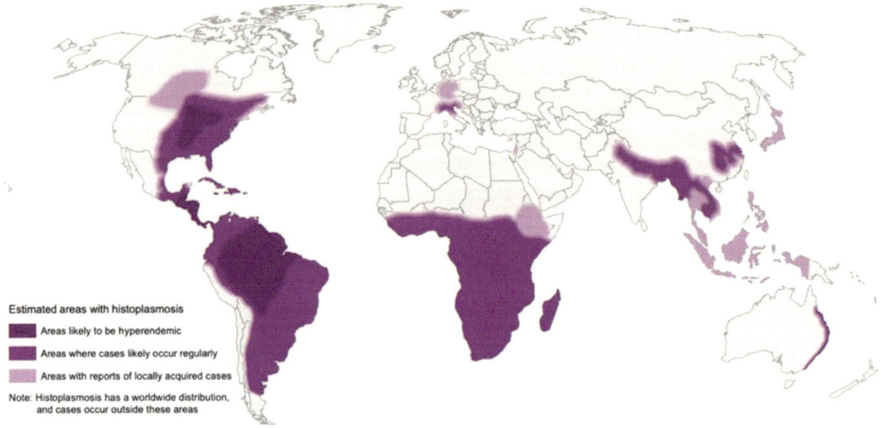

Figure 5.
World map estimating regions most likely to have histoplasmosis based on literature review (2020) [94]. https://link.springer.com/article/10.1007/s11046-020-00431-2.

reported in the remained continents, except Antarctica. Recently, the fungus has been detected in soil and penguin droppings even in the Antarctic peninsula [39].

The geographic distribution of *H. capsulatum* in the North America remains still unclear and requires further investigations [100].

In highly endemic areas around the US river valleys, population skin delayed type hypersensitivity to histoplasmin is around 90%, meaning that residents of these areas were exposed to the primary infection at some point in their lifetime [16, 69].

In most of them the infection is inapparent, asymptomatic and only less than 1% of them will develop the disease [101].

Extrapolating these figures to the entire population, nearly 50 million Americans are latently infected with *H. capsulatum* [16]. Epidemiological reports and studies have shown many cases of histoplasmosis diagnosed in humans or animals outside historically recognized endemic areas. The distribution of these cases extends beyond the originally defined boundaries of the US river valleys [43, 94], encompassing states in the north (Minnesota, Wisconsin, Michigan), northeast (New York), and west (California, Arizona, Idaho, and Montana) [74].

However, the real picture of Histoplasma geographic distribution, potential exposure, and relevant host factors is still incomplete in the USA, histoplasmosis not being part of the diseases with mandatory national notification, being voluntary reported only in 13 states. These states do not necessarily include the relevant ones where histoplasmosis has traditionally been diagnosed. A recent CDC report summarizes 2019 US surveillance data on histoplasmosis and confirmed that Histoplasma causes substantial illness in the USA, with the high rates of hospitalization and death. Reported data rely on the national case definition established in 2017 by the Council of State and Territory Epidemiologists (CSTE), which classifies histoplasmosis cases as confirmed or probable based on laboratory, and clinical and epidemiological criteria. The findings showed that the overall incidence of histoplasmosis was 1.8 cases per 100,000 population, 54% of patients were hospitalized, and 5% died. Three northeastern states were accountable for 65% of the cases: Minnesota (19%) with an incidence rate of 3.8, and Michigan (20%) and Illinois (26%) with a rate of 3.2 each [93]. Using county-level data on histoplasmosis cases reported between 2011 and 2014 in 12 states (covering the eastern half of the USA), a recent estimate from 2022 supports the hypothesis of a shift in the presence of *H. capsulatum* toward the northeastern and central states around the Great Lakes and the Atlantic coast [100].

In a retrospective study performed between 2002 and 2017 in PLHIV in the USA, the overall mortality rate proved to be 37% with an early mortality of 14.8% and late mortality of 22.2%, with no statistically significant difference in survival in those treated with HAART [102].

In the USA, there are estimated 25,000 cases of life-threatening Histoplasma infections [18] and over 5000 histoplasmosis-related hospitalizations annually [70, 87]. Between 2001 and 2012, the proportion of histoplasmosis-related hospitalizations in people with diabetes, transplanted or receiving biologic agents had increased, while in people living with HIV/ AIDS had decreased from 21.5% to 17.3%. The mean length of histoplasmosis-associated hospitalizations is almost double compared with that non-histoplasmosis related. In 2012, the total burden for histoplasmosis-related hospitalizations was estimated at $371 million [70].

In Canada, histoplasmosis is considered endemic in the regions adjacent to the St. Lawrence River and the Great Lakes, especially Quebec and Ontario. A northward expansion of the disease has been observed, evidenced by a continued increase (0.05 to 0.25 per 100,000 people) in confirmed cases of histoplasmosis in Alberta between 1990 and 2015 [43, 94, 103].

Histoplasmosis is endemic in Central and South America [94], excepting the western part of the two continents (west Mexico and Peru, and most of Chile) [43]. Histoplasmin skin test sensitivity average is 32% in the general population of Latin America [94]. High-endemicity areas are Guatemala, Brazil, Venezuela, Ecuador, Uruguay, Paraguay, and Argentina [16].

The variability of histoplasmin test results is high in the states of Latin America, with rates of nearly 90% in Guatemala, some areas of Mexico [69] and Southeastern Brazil, 63% in Midwestern Brazil [16], 42% in Trinidad and Tobago and Venezuela, and 37% in Costa Rica and Nicaragua [94].

Histoplasmosis is an increasing challenge for the Latin American population, especially the disseminated form of the disease occurring in HIV-positive patients [68]. In PLHIV histoplasmosis is as widespread as tuberculosis [94]. Some studies estimate more than 15,000 new histoplasmosis cases occurring annually [104] and up to 30% mortality rate [105].

In a large prospective cohort study, conducted in Guatemala between 2005 and 2009, which enrolled HIV-positive patients with suspected histoplasmosis, crude mortality in patients with histoplasmosis was 43.6 versus 30.8% among no-histoplasmosis patients. Also, early mortality rate was 24.8% among histoplasmosis cases, statistically significantly higher than non-histoplasmosis ones (9.3%). Coinfection with *Mycobacterium tuberculosis* was found in 9.9% of patients [106], data which is similar with other findings from some Latin America countries where mycobacterial coinfection was reported in 8% (in French Guiana) to 15% (Panama) of HIV+ patients with Histoplasma infection [107].

Interestingly, patients infected with Histoplasma alone had lower survival rates than those coinfected with Histoplasma and *M. tuberculosis* [106].

A robust study of more than 58% of the newly diagnosed HIV patients, reported by the national HIV program during 2017–2018, in Guatemala found that histoplasmosis was the most common opportunistic infection, with an overall incidence of 7.9%, varying from 1.1 to 19.7% in patients with CD4 cell counts higher than 350 cells/mm^3 and lower than 50 cells/mm^3, respectively. Of all patients enrolled, 18.1% had opportunistic infections, of which 36.4% was histoplasmosis. In those with two underlying opportunistic infections, histoplasmosis was frequently associated with cryptococcal disease and tuberculosis in 35.5 and 32.3% of cases, respectively. Mortality rates in disseminated histoplasmosis were significantly statistical higher than in non-disseminated cases (32.7 versus 13.3%) [108].

A screening program for histoplasmosis in HIV-positive patients in Guatemala showed an increasing trend in the number of newly diagnosed cases of histoplasmosis, with the annual incidence rising from 6.5% in 2017 to 8.8% in 2019. As a result of early diagnosis and rapid initiation of treatment, 180-day mortality rates showed an annual downward trend, from 32.8% in 2017 to 21.2% in 2019, underscoring the importance of implementing screening programs in endemic areas and populations at risk for decreasing mortality [109].

In a cohort of HIV-infected patients from French Guiana followed between 2010 and 2019, disseminated histoplasmosis was the most common opportunistic infection with an early case fatality rate of 3.9 within 1 month of diagnosis. It is important to emphasize that the analysis of the evolution of histoplasmosis cases showed that as diagnosis rates improved and, consequently due to treatment, the huge early fatality rate (40%) from 1992 to 1997 decreased more than 10 times in this cohort, leading to better outcomes in most patients with disseminated form of disease [110].

A systematic review of 3530 published cases of disease and isolates of *H. capsulatum* from environmental and animal sources between 1939 and 2018 in Brazil showed that histoplasmosis is endemic throughout Brazil, especially in Northeastern, Central-Western Southeastern, and Southern areas. Disseminated histoplasmosis was the prevalent form of disease, described in more than 80% of reported cases in Brazil. The main underlying condition was HIV infection, found in 97.2% of patients with immunosuppression. Coinfection with *M. tuberculosis* was found in 10.37% patients, these findings being like those found in Guatemala and other Latin American countries. Mortality rate was 33.1% [111]. The north-eastern state of Brazil, the estate of Ceará, is a highly endemic area of histoplasmosis, with many disseminated histoplasmosis cases in people living with HIV, being considered the area with the highest mortality rate due to histoplasmosis (33–42%) [45, 112].

Genetic diversity among isolates and sexual reproduction of *H. capsulatum* in Brazilian population support the hypothesis that Brazil is the center of origin of Histoplasma spp. in Latin America, most likely with the contribution of migratory birds and bats [52].

On African continent, despite the significant number of people living with HIV, histoplasmosis remains an underdiagnosed and neglected disease. The lack of skin tests surveys necessary to develop a much more detailed geographic understanding of the distribution of the disease has impeded the clear delimitation of areas of hyperendemicity.

An exhaustive review on histoplasmosis cases reported from 32 African countries between 1952 and 2017, performed by Oladele and her colleagues, reveals a comprehensive picture of the disease distribution across the continent. Both varieties of *H. capsulatum* coexist in the African territory, *H. capsulatum* var. capsulatum (Hcc) being found predominantly in Southern and Northern Africa and *H. capsulatum* var. duboisii (Hcd) being prevalent in the West, Central, and East of the continent. Moreover, Hcc is found mostly in HIV-positive adults, while Hcd is reported especially in immunocompetent children [113]. Although less common in the African AIDS patients, Hcd is more likely to produce the disseminated form of the disease [94, 113] with a case fatality rate around 23% [65].

The disease is more prevalent in Western Africa (especially Nigeria), Southern Africa (South Africa and Zimbabwe), and Central-Eastern countries (Congo, Uganda) with a nonuniform distribution of isolated cases in many other states across the continent [94, 113].

Of the total number of cases reported in Africa, Nigeria accounts for more than a quarter (26.4%), all exclusively involving Hcd and, with an overwhelming majority (96.7%), in HIV-negative patients [113]. Interestingly, Nigeria has high variable rate in the histoplasmin reactivity test between rural (35%) and urban areas (4.4%) [94, 113].

Hcc was the exclusive causative microorganism, affecting almost equally the HIV-positive and the negative population in South Africa, which had 13% of the cases of histoplasmosis in Africa. In Zimbabwe, the percentage of cases was 12% of mainland cases, diagnosed exclusively in HIV-positive patients, all but one caused by Hcc [113].

The prognosis of disseminated histoplasmosis in Africa is poor, fatality rates varying between 23% for *H. capsulatum* var. duboisii and 50% for *H. capsulatum* var. capsulatum infections [84, 114, 115].

Within Asia, histoplasmosis is endemic in China, especially along the Yangtze River [116], Thailand, South Korea, and India [17].

A study of hospitalized patients and healthy residents in China found overall values of histoplasmin reactivity of 9.0%, with higher values in Jiangsu province (15.1%) [117].

In Sichuan Province, histoplasmin test positivity was found between 21.8% in healthy adults and 28.6% in hospitalized TB patients [118].

A review of 300 cases of histoplasmosis recorded in China between 1990 and 2011 found three quarters of cases in southeastern territory, along the Yangtze River. More than 85% were patients with disseminated histoplasmosis, most of them with underlying immunocompromising conditions such as HIV infection, diabetes, and liver disease [116].

A study of 4211 lifelong residents of Thailand found uneven distribution in the 8 regions studied, with histoplasmin sensitivity ranging from rates of 4.8% in the north and northeast to 34.4% in the south and center, which are among the highest reported in Asia. Due to the endemicity of Talaromyces marneffei in the region, the hypothesis of overestimation of the sensitivity to histoplasmin through cross-reactivity with this fungal antigen was issued [119].

In Thailand, histoplasmosis is reportable to the Ministry of Public Health, and between 1984 and 2010, a total of 1253 cases were documented among exclusively patients living with HIV in this country [120].

In Myanmar, a study of histoplasmin skin test sensitivity in prisoners and their families showed rates ranging from 8.4 to 27.1% [98, 121].

Cases of histoplasmosis have also been reported in other Southeast Asian countries, where histoplasmin reactivity ranges from 2.7–63.6% in Indonesia, 11.8% in Malaysia, 33.7% in Vietnam, and 6.4–26% in the Philippines, supporting the hypothesis of the endemicity of histoplasmosis in these areas [94, 98].

Histoplasma has been known to be present in India for many years since it was first reported to be present in the soil of Gangetic Plain in 1975 [122]. Most cases of histoplasmosis were reported in north-eastern areas, especially West Bengal and Assam states, crossed by the Ganges, Yamuna, and Brahmaputra Rivers. Yet, it is very likely that the number of cases is underestimated, due to misdiagnosis as tuberculosis or leishmaniasis [123, 124]. The histoplasmin test positivity rate reported in a study between 1950 and 1970 was 12.3% in northern India [125].

In a retrospective analysis of cases published between 2001 and 2015, it was found that most of them were reported in the north-eastern part of India, six times more frequently in men than in women, and were associated with agricultural activity. Patients with underlying immunocompromising conditions were around 33% of cases, of which HIV infection was the main cause of immunosuppression. The mortality rate was 27.5% in immunosuppressed versus 10% in immunocompetent patients with histoplasmosis [124].

In Japan, histoplasmosis is rarely reported, and most diagnosed cases are considered imported from endemic areas [44]. A study on 187 bat guano samples collected from 67 bat-inhabited caves in Japan was unable to detect *H. capsulatum*, by either method [126].

Isolated and scattered cases of locally acquired histoplasmosis have been reported since 1948 in all Australian states except Tasmania. Endemic areas are Queensland and northern New South Wales, regions traversed by the long Dumaresq and Macintyre rivers. In a report of cases and literature review of cases in Australia, 41% of disseminated form was found in HIV infected patients. The prognosis of patients with disseminated disease was poor, this form being associated with a 30% recurrence rate and a 37% mortality rate [99].

Europe is a non-endemic area for histoplasmosis, and the disease is rarely reported and is considered a predominantly imported disease. The majority of cases are linked to travel in endemic areas or immigration [127].

In a review of 118 cases of histoplasmosis diagnosed in Europe between 1995 and 1999, more than 93% of patients had a history of migration or travel to a known endemic area. The remaining 6.8% were considered autochthonous European cases, and these patients having no travel history outside their country of origin (Italy, Turkey, and Germany). Notably in this survey, cases of disseminated histoplasmosis were diagnosed among elderly residents of the United Kingdom who fought in India and Myanmar during World War II and who had not left their country of origin for over 50 years after returning from the war. Out of 8 non-imported cases, Italy was the country with the most cases diagnosed as autochthonous [128]. This is consistent with the isolation of *H. capsulatum* in the soil [129] and dogs [130] in the Po Valley area in Italy and with the histoplasmin positivity rate of 1.2% in the population of this area. Few sporadic cases of autochthonous histoplasmosis have also been described in Spain [131].

A more recent systematic review of histoplasmosis cases in the literature identified 223 patients diagnosed between 2005 and 2020 in 17 European countries and Israel. Only eight cases were classified as autochthonous (four in Italy, two in Spain, one in Ireland, and one in Israel), the remaining majority of 96.4% being imported, especially from Latin America and Sub-Saharan Africa. More than 64% of imported cases of histoplasmosis were diagnosed in 3 European countries: Spain (36.7%), France (19.5%), and Italy (7.9%). The other countries reporting the remaining cases of imported histoplasmosis were the Netherland, Germany, Switzerland, United Kingdom, Poland, Austria, Slovenia, Portugal, Greece, Ireland, Sweden, Belgium, Finland, Denmark, and Israel. Most of the cases were recorded in HIV-infected patients (over 51.1%), in whom progressive disseminated histoplasmosis was the most common form of clinical presentation (89.47%). The patients with other immunocompromising diseases were 12.5%, histoplasmosis manifesting in its disseminated form in 57.1% of these cases. In a smaller percentage (6.2%), the picture of progressive disseminated histoplasmosis was also encountered in immunocompetent individuals. The worst outcome of histoplasmosis (32% mortality rate) was registered in patients with other than HIV underlying immunocompromised conditions, while in patients living with HIV infection the mortality rate was 24.3% [132].

In conclusion, doctors from non-endemic areas must consider in certain cases the differential diagnosis with histoplasmosis in immunosuppressed patients and especially in those with HIV infection, because early diagnosis and rapid institution of therapy improve the outcome of the disease and patient's survival [97].

4. Pathogenesis

In most cases, the onset of infection occurs *via* inhalation of airborne microconidia or mycelial fragments of *H. capsulatum* [133]. The portal of entry are the lungs, the fungus bypassing the innate defenses of the host (muco-ciliary clearance, nasal and pharyngeal mucus, and pulmonary surfactant) and reaching the terminal bronchioles and pulmonary alveoli [54].

Shortly after it was inhaled, triggered by the body temperature, it undergoes the dimorphic switching to the budding yeast form within hours and is deposited in macrophages [64].

It may happen that the conidia enter the alveolar macrophages and become yeast there, or the transition occurs first and then the yeast enters the macrophages.

Fungus internalization into the macrophages is determined by a couple of specific immune evasive mechanisms: i.) Histoplasma maximizes macrophages recognition through heat shock protein 60 kDa (HSP60), which mediates the fungal detection and binding by the CD18 integrin family of receptors, on the surface of the macrophages [62, 64]. ii.) Concomitantly, *H. capsulatum* minimizes detection of immunostimulatory β-glucans by Dectin-1 receptors of dendritic cells both by synthetizing an α-(1,3)-glucan layer covering its β-glucans upper layer and by secreting endoglucanase, which enzymatically removes the remained uncovered, still exposed β-glucans. Once internalized, *H. capsulatum* resides in the phagosome compartment without fusing with the lysosome, displaying several pathogenic mechanisms, and thus blocking normal phagosome maturation process in macrophages One of these mechanisms consists in alkalinization of the phagosome and phagolysosome, maintaining the pH between 6.0 and 6.5, which both inhibit the normal function of lysosomal hydrolases and maximize iron acquisition from the host transferrin. Other required strategies for growing and proliferation within nutrient-depleted phagosome compartment are the following: expressing antioxidant enzymes (superoxide dismutase 3 Sod3 and catalase B CatB) that eliminate reactive oxygen intermediates [63, 134], expressing enzymes involved in gluconeogenesis for providing energy and glucans, using amino acids as carbon, nitrogen, and sulfur sources, acquisition of essential vitamins, and trace metals (iron, zinc, and copper) [134].

Thereby, macrophages are not only ineffective in neutralizing *H. capsulatum* yeast but, on the contrary, serve the pathogen by creating a hospitable intracellular niche, in which it can unabatedly multiply and survive [62]. The intracellular deposition and proliferation of the fungus varies, depending on the yeast elements and the host cells; at some point, the multiplied yeast cells destroy the macrophage and are ingested both by new other alveolar macrophages and by other phagocytic cells recruited at the site of infection [135].

During the next 2 weeks after inhalation, when specific immunity develops [136], macrophages also act as vehicles, initially in spreading the fungus to hilar and mediastinal lymph nodes and later in hematogenous dissemination of infection to multiple organs [137].

Besides the macrophages, which are the main host cells for *H. capsulatum* [64], other host defense cells, including dendritic cells and neutrophils, are recruited at the locus of infection and interact with the fungus [62].

By releasing their azurophilic granule contents, neutrophils can inhibit *H. capsulatum* growth. In the case of a small inoculum, it has been hypothesized that this fungistatic activity of neutrophils could be sufficient to cleanse the host, without triggering the subsequent mechanisms of the adaptive immune response [138].

Dendritic cells engulf some yeast cells, *via* fibronectin receptors, and are capable to kill them, thus releasing nucleic acids of the destroyed yeasts, and recovering presentable antigens [62].

These immune responses combined with dendritic cells production of proinflammatory TNF, IL-6, IL-12, and type I interferons (IFN-I) stimulate activation of $CD4^+$ lymphocytes [62, 139]. Once activated, this specific adaptive immune response can either clear the infection or cause the formation of epithelioid granulomas [54], with later evolution toward fibrosis and calcification, mimicking tuberculosis [97].

Like Mycoplasma tuberculosis, *H. capsulatum* could remain dormant, in a quiescent state in this fibrotic tissue, even for decades, and reactivate when cell-mediated immunity is impaired by other diseases or immunosuppressive therapies [54, 68, 97].

Additionally, in situations where T helper lymphocytes are low or even absent, as might be found in severely immunosuppressed patients, dendritic cells can activate $CD8^+$ cells, by cross-presenting them *H. capsulatum* antigen acquired from apoptotic macrophages [140]. In these cases, the granuloma formation is almost absent, the proliferation of macrophages occurring in the tissues, and the patients tend to develop progressive, disseminated form of disease [97].

Although humoral immunity has an unclear role in the pathogenesis of histoplasmosis, depletion of B cells has nevertheless been shown to increase the severity of histoplasmosis, while experimental treatments with monoclonal antibodies to *H. capsulatum* surface antigens have been beneficial in disease evolution in mice [16].

In conclusion, T lymphocytes and phagocytes are essential cellular elements of *H. capsulatum* pathogenesis, the outcome of infection being orchestrated by the dynamics between innate and adaptive host responses and yeast virulence factors [61, 141].

5. Prevention and prophylaxis

5.1 Non-pharmacologic strategies for prevention

People with occupations or hobbies that involve outdoor activities associated with soil aerosolization and exposure to guano for birds or bats, agricultural and forestry workers, fishermen or hunters, and people employed in construction have a 5–10 times higher risk than from the general population [66].

To reduce the risk of illness in immunosuppressed patients living in areas endemic for histoplasmosis, the CDC recommends protective measures: avoid disturbing soil contaminated with chicken or bird guano or cleaning chicken coops, demolishing, remodeling, renovate or cleaning buildings, exploring caves, tunnels, or old archeological sites.

To minimize the risk of infection with *H. capsulatum* at the workplace, concrete measures are needed that can be identified by applying the control hierarchy framework used by health and safety at work specialists. Thus, the following measures are required:

- preventing the accumulation of bird or bat droppings and excluding bats or birds from a building by sealing all entry and exit points, installing lights in daytime roost areas, building bat houses near former roosts, using of visual and auditory deterrents, the periodic application of non-toxic chemical substances to repel birds, and the installation of mechanical anti-bird roosting systems;

- controlling dust generation and aerosolized dust by spraying the dry material with water, adding a surfactant or wetting agent to the water, using an industrial vacuum cleaner with a filter to collect the contaminated material, using bulldozers that have air-conditioned cabs and HEPA filtration, covering the bed of trucks carrying dirt or debris from a construction site, and washing the trucks before leaving the construction site;

- disinfecting potentially contaminated material using formaldehyde is no longer recommended because it causes a variety of health problems and there are no approved products registered specifically as soil disinfectants or as being effective against Histoplasma;

- administrative controls by publication of health risk warnings displayed in areas known or suspected to be contaminated with Histoplasma and by training workers on potential workplace hazards and associated safety practices, procedures, and safeguards;

- wearing personal protective equipment (PPE) to protect employees from Histoplasma contamination by using respirators equipped with filters or masks, safety glasses, disposable protective clothing, and covering shoes or boots.

The hierarchy of controls can also be used to prevent worker exposure to *H. capsulatum* in laboratory environments by: knowledge of the laboratory safety manual, training of laboratory personnel, medical supervision, through aseptic microbiological practices, handling of clinical and culture samples in a biosafety level (BSL)-3 laboratory and a laminar flow Biological Safety Cabinet (BSC) with wearing appropriate PPE, packing or taping closed culture plates, not performing slide cultures, and testing with molecular and proteomic approaches.

Including systematic collection of occupational information as part of histoplasmosis surveillance could facilitate the identification of future workplace-associated outbreaks and the identification of specific risk factors that require further evaluation [66].

5.2 Specific prevention

To date, there is no immunization option available to prevent or treat any fungal infection. Although there have been numerous attempts to develop a potential vaccine against histoplasmosis, these candidates have only been tested on murine models. Various strategies have been used in the search for an effective vaccine for histoplasmosis. The active immunization approaches used in the research consisted of administration of recombinant heat shock protein rHsp60 or only the small protein fragment F3 of rHsp60, the surface protein H antigen, or auto-transplantation into a murine model of dendritic cells, primed *in vitro*, with apoptotic macrophages obtained by phagocytizing *H. capsulatum* yeast, inactivated by heat.

Research studies based on passive immunization methods have focused on the administration of monoclonal antibodies (mAbs Ig.M against histone 2B, mAbs Ig.G against rHsp60) or therapeutic pan-anti-fungal antibodies.

Immune system modulation strategies targeting the programmed cell death receptor-1 (PD-1) and its ligand (PD-L) have suggested that selective blockade of the PD-1/PD-L pathway may play a key therapeutic role in fungal immunity, not only for histoplasmosis but also for other mycoses [142].

The latest research in this field, approaching revolutionary methods of reverse vaccinology, comparative genomics, and molecular docking, have identified some candidate targets to produce both vaccines and new drugs against *H. capsulatum*. The most promising candidate vaccine target appears to be beta-1,3-glucanosyl transferase, the enzyme involved in the elongation of beta-(1-3)-glucans in the fungal cell wall, but further *in vivo* research is needed to test its efficacy and safety [143].

Recently, the WHO has released the fungal priority pathogen list (FPPL) to strengthen the global response against fungal infections. The FPPL highlights the need for actions, interventions, and strategies that focus on three main areas: surveillance, research and development, and public health actions [40].

5.3 Prophylaxis

Prophylactic use of antifungal drugs has been studied only in persons with HIV infection [48]. A placebo-controlled trial showed that primary prophylaxis with itraconazole capsules prevents histoplasmosis in patients living with HIV infection, and even a survival benefit was not demonstrated [144].

Prophylaxis of histoplasmosis with 200 mg daily of itraconazole should be considered only in patients with HIV infection with CD4 cell counts <150 cells/ mm^3, in highly endemic areas in which the incidence of the disease is higher than 10 cases per 100 patient-years (A-I evidence-based recommendation).

In other immunosuppressed patients, daily prophylaxis with itraconazole may be appropriate, in specific circumstances (C-III). There are no data on the role and appropriate duration for prophylaxis in a patient who is receiving immunosuppressive therapy for organ transplantation, malignancy, or chronic inflammatory disease and who, concomitantly, exhibits radiographic or serologic evidence of past histoplasmosis [19]. On the other hand, the risk for histoplasmosis appears to be low in patients receiving immunosuppressive therapy for solid organ or bone marrow transplantation, with an estimated incidence less than 1%, even in endemic areas [145]. For patients receiving therapy with TNF antagonists, there is a risk for developing the disseminated form of the disease, histoplasmosis being considered the most common fungal infection associated with this treatment [146]. History of active histoplasmosis in the last 2 years could be considered a benchmark for initiating prophylaxis with itraconazole during immunosuppression. Also, patients who have finished treatment for histoplasmosis and who are about to receive a transplant or to start new immunosuppressive therapies should be tested for the levels of urinary histoplasma antigen before the intervention and then every 2 or 3 months after. An increase in urinary antigen levels indicates the need for further investigation for active histoplasmosis, but a consistent elevation of the urinary histoplasma antigen level should prompt empirically initiation of antifungal therapy, in the context of ongoing immunosuppression [19].

Transplacental transmission of *H. capsulatum* to the fetus [146] could be prevented by administering antifungal therapy before delivery, but there are no evidence-based guidelines for the management of the vertical mode of transmission. Histopathological examination of the placenta for granuloma and for other organisms resembling *H. capsulatum* should be performed [19].

6. Conclusion

Histoplasma infections are more widespread than traditionally appreciated, mainly due to misdiagnosis in some regions or diagnostic and therapeutic deficiencies in others. Expanding surveillance and case reporting would provide a more accurate picture for a better understanding of the geographic distribution of histoplasmosis. The disease remains an important factor in morbidity and mortality in many parts of the world.

Conflict of interest

The authors declare no conflict of interest.

Author details

Nela Daniela Efrim[1*], Elena Dumea[2,3] and Roxana Carmen Cernat[1]

1 Faculty of Medicine, "Ovidius" University of Constanta, Romania, Infectious Diseases Hospital, Constanta, Romania

2 4th Department - Clinical Medical Disciplines, Faculty of Medicine, 'Ovidius' University of Constanta, Constanta, Romania

3 Clinical Infectious Disease Hospital, Constanta, Romania

*Address all correspondence to: daniela.efrim@gmail.com

References

[1] Hawksworth DL. The fungal dimension of biodiversity: Magnitude, significance, and conservation. Mycological Research. 1991;**95**:641-655. DOI: 10.1016/S0953-7562(09)80810-1

[2] Hawksworth DL, Lücking R. Fungal diversity revisited: 2.2 to 3.8 million species. Microbiology Spectrum. 2017;**5**(4). Article number: FUNK-0052-2016. DOI: 10.1128/microbiolspec.FUNK-0052-2016

[3] Blackwell M. The fungi: 1,2,3...5.1 million species? American Journal of Botany. 2011;**98**(3):426-438. DOI: 103732/ajb.1000298

[4] Van Rhijn N, Bromley M. The consequences of our changing environment on life threatening and debilitating fungal disease in humans. Journal of Fungi. 2021;**7**(5):367-384. DOI: 10.3390/jof7050367

[5] Hyde KD. The numbers of fungi. Fungal Diversity. 2022;**114**:1. DOI: 10.1007/s13225-022-00507-y

[6] Phukhamsakda C, Nilsson RH, Bhunjun CS, Gomes de Faria AR, Sun Y, Wijesinghe SN, et al. The numbers of fungi: Contributions from traditional taxonomic studies and challenges of metabarcoding. Fungal diversity. 2022;**114**:327-386. DOI: 10.1007/s13225-022-00502-3

[7] Xu J. Assessing global fungal threats to humans. mLife. 2022;**1**:223-240. DOI: 10.1002/mlf2.12036

[8] Cheek M, Nic Lughadha E, Kirk P, Lindon H, Carretero J, Looney B, et al. New scientific discoveries: Plants and fungi. Plants, People, Planet. 2020;**2**:371-388. DOI: 10.1002/ppp3.10148

[9] Richardson MD. Changing patterns and trends in systemic fungal infections. Journal of Antimicrobial Chemotherapy. 2005;**56**(1):i5-i11. DOI: 10.1093/jac/dki218

[10] Fisher MC, Gow NAR, Gurr SJ. Tackling emerging fungal threats to animal health, food security and ecosystem resilience. Philosophical Transactions of the Royal Society B: Biological Sciences. 2016;**371**:20160332. DOI: 10.1098/rstb.2016.0332

[11] Gow NAR, Netea MG. Medical mycology and fungal immunology: New research perspectives addressing a major world health challenge. Philosophical Transactions of the Royal Society B: Biological Sciences. 2016;**371**:20150462. DOI: 10.1098/rstb.2015.0462

[12] Bongomin F, Gago S, Oladele RO, Denning DW. Global and multinational prevalence of fungal diseases-estimate precision. Journal of Fungi. 2017;**3**(4):57. DOI: 10.3390/jof3040057

[13] de Hoog GS, Chaturvedi V, Denning DW, Dyer PS, Frisvad JC, Geiser D, et al. Name changes in medically important fungi and their implications for clinical practice. Journal of Clinical Microbiology. 2015;**53**(4):1056-1062. DOI: 10.1128/JCM.02016-14

[14] de Hoog GS, Guarro J, Gené J, Ahmed S, Al-Hatmi AMS, Figueras MJ, et al. Atlas of Clinical Fungi. 4th ed. Hilversum: Foundation Atlas of Clinical Fungi. 2020. p. 1599

[15] Köhler JR, Hube B, Puccia R, Casadevall A, Perfect JR. Fungi that infect humans. Microbiology Spectrum. 2017;**5**(3):5.3.08. DOI: 10.1128/microbiolspec.FUNK-0014-2016

[16] Taborda CP, Buccheri R, Benard G, Duarte-Neto AN, Nosanchuk JD, Travassos LR. Paracoccidioides spp. and *Histoplasma capsulatum*: Current and new perspectives for diagnosis and treatment. Current Topics in Medicinal Chemistry. 2018;**18**(15):1333-1348. DOI: 10.2174/1568026618666181002112231

[17] Valdez AF, Miranda DZ, Guimarães AJ, Nimrichter L, Nosanchuk JD. Pathogenicity and virulence of *Histoplasma capsulatum* - a multifaceted organism adapted to intracellular environments. Virulence. 2022;**13**(1):1900-1919. DOI: 10.1080/21505594.2022.2137987

[18] Brown GD, Denning DW, Gow NAR, Levitz SM, Netea MG, White TC. Hidden killers: Human fungal infections. Science Translational Medicine. 2012;**4**(165):165rv13. DOI: 10.1126/scitranslmed.3004404

[19] Wheat LJ, Freifeld AG, Kleiman MB, Baddley JW, McKinsey DS, Loyd JE, et al. IDSA clinical practice guidelines for the management of patients with histoplasmosis: 2007 update by the infectious disease society of America. Clinical Infectious Disease. 2007;**45**(7):807-825. DOI: 10.1086/521259

[20] Cano MV, Hajjeh RA. The epidemiology of histoplasmosis: A review. Seminars in Respiratory Infections. 2001;**16**(2):109-118. DOI: 10.1053/srin.2001.24241

[21] Darling ST. A protozoon general infection producing pseudotubercles in the lungs and focal necroses in the liver, spleen and lymphnodes. Journal of the American Medical Association. 1906;**46**:1283-1285. DOI: 10.1001/JAMA.1906.62510440037003

[22] Conant NF. Cultural study of the life cycle of *Histoplasma capsulatum* Darling 1906. Journal of Bacteriology. 1941;**41**(5):563-579. DOI: 10.1128/jb.41.5.563-579.1941

[23] Dodd K, Tompkins EH. A case of histoplasmosis of Darling in a infant. American Journal of Tropical Medicine. 1934;**14**:127-137

[24] Zarafonetis CJD, Lindberg RB. Histoplasmosis of Darling. Observations on antigenic properties of causative agent. Preliminary report. University Hospital Ann Arbor. 1941;7:47-48

[25] Duncan JT. A unique form of Histoplasma. Transactions of the Royal Society of Tropical Medicine and Hygiene. 1947;**40**(4):364

[26] Mochi A, Edwards PQ. Geographical distribution of histoplasmosis and histoplasmin sensitivity. Bulletin World Health Organization. 1952;**5**(3):259-291

[27] Christie A, Peterson JC. Pulmonary calcifications in negative reactors to tuberculin. American Journal of Public Health and the Nation's Health. 1945;**35**(11):1131-1147. DOI: 10.2105/ajph.35.11.1131

[28] Palmer CE. Nontuberculous pulmonary calcifications and sensitivity to histoplasmin. Public Health Reports. 1945;**60**:513-520

[29] Arblaster PG. Pulmonary histoplasmosis. Thorax. 1950;**5**:333-339

[30] Emmons CW. Isolation of *Histoplasma capsulatum* from soil. Public Health Reports. 1949;**64**(28):892-896

[31] Dubois A, Janssens PG, Brutsaert P, Vanbreuseghem R. A case of African histoplasmosis; with a mycological note on Histoplasma duboisii n. sp. Annales de la Societe belge de medicine tropicale. 1952;**32**(6):569-584

[32] Edwards LB, Acquaviva FA, Livesay VT, Cross FW, Palmer CE. An atlas of sensitivity to tuberculin, PPD-B, and histoplasmin in the United States. The American Review of Respiratory Disease. 1969;**99**(4):1-132

[33] Kwon-Chung KJ. Sexual stage of *Histoplasma capsulatum*. Science. 1972;**175**(4019):326. DOI: 10.1126/science.175.4019.326

[34] Kwon-Chung KJ. Emmonsilla capsulata: Perfect state of *Histoplasma capsulatum*. Science. 1972;**177**(4046):368-369. DOI: 10.1126/science.177.4046.368

[35] Hwang L, Hocking-Murray D, Bahrami AK, Andesson M, Rine J, Sil A. Identifying phase-specific genes in the fungal pathogen *Histoplasma capsulatum* using a genomic shotgun microarray. Molecular Biology of the Cell. 2003;**14**(6):2314-2326. DOI: 10.1091/mbc.e03-01-0027

[36] Kasuga T, White TJ, Koenig G, McEwen J, Restrepo A, Castañeda E, et al. Phylogeography of the fungal pathogen *Histoplasma capsulatum*. Molecular Ecology. 2003;**12**(12):3383-3401. DOI: 10.1046/j.1365-294x.2003.01995.x

[37] Whitt SP, Koch GA, Fender B, Ratnasamy N, Everett ED. Histoplasmosis in pregnancy: Case series and report of transplacental transmission. Archives of Internal Medicine. 2004;**164**(4):454-458. DOI: 10.1001/archinte.164.4.454

[38] Damasceno LS, Vite-Garín T, Ramírez JA, Rodríguez-Arellanes G, Almeida MAD, Muniz MDM, et al. Mixed infection by *Histoplasma capsulatum* isolates with different mating types in Brazilian AIDS-patients. Revista do Instituto de Medicina Tropical de São Paulo. 2019;**61**. Article number: e8. DOI: 10.1590/s1678-9946201961008

[39] Moreira LM, Meyer W, Chame M, Brandão LM, Vivoni AM, Portugal J, et al. Molecular detection of *Histoplasma capsulatum* in Antarctica. Emerging Infectious Diseases. 2022;**28**(10):2100-2104. DOI: 10.3201/eid2810.220046

[40] The WHO lists multiple fungal pathogens of critical, high and medium importance for addressing with R&D, surveillance and access to diagnosis and treatment. 2022. Available from: https://gaffi.org/wp-content/uploads/WHO-FPPL-2022.pdf. [Accessed: 2023-03-03]

[41] Beyhan S, Sil A. Sensing the heat and the host: Virulence determinants of *Histoplasma capsulatum*. Virulence. 2019;**10**:793-800. DOI: 10.1080/21505594.2019.1663596

[42] Edwards JA, Rappleye CA. Histoplasma mechanisms of pathogenesis - one portfolio doesn't fit all. FEMS Microbiology Letters. 2011;**324**:1-9. DOI: 10.1111/j.1574-6968.2011.02363.x

[43] Lockhart SR, Toda M, Benedict K, Caceres DH, Litvintseva AP. Endemic and other dimorphic mycoses in the Americas. Journal of Fungi. 2021;7(2):151. DOI: 10.3390/jof7020151

[44] Scully MC, Baddley JW. Epidemiology of histoplasmosis. Current Fungal Infection Reports. 2018;**12**:51-58. DOI: 10.1007/s12281-018-0309-x

[45] Damasceno LS, Teixeira MM, Barker BM, Almeida MA, Muniz MM, Pizzini CV, et al. Novel clinical and dual infection by *Histoplasma capsulatum* genotypes in HIV patients from Northeastern, Brazil. Scientific Reports. 2019;**9**(1):11789. DOI: 10.1038/s41598-019-48111-6

[46] Diaz JH. Environmental and wilderness-related risk factors for

histoplasmosis: More than bats in caves. Wilderness & Environmental Medicine. 2018;**29**(4):531-540. DOI: 10.1016/j.wem.2018.06.008

[47] Vite-Garín T, Estrada-Bárcenas DA, Cifuentes J, Taylor ML. The importance of molecular analyses for understanding the genetic diversity of *Histoplasma Capsulatum*: An overview. Revista Iberoamericana de Micología. 2014;**31**(1):11-15. DOI: 10.1016/j.riam.2013.09.013

[48] Kauffman CA. Histoplasmosis. In: Kauffman CA, Pappas PG, Sobel JD, Dismukes WE, editors. Essentials of Clinical Mycology. 2nd ed. New-York: Springer Science + Business Media LLC; 2011. pp. 321-336. DOI: 10.1007/978-1-4419-6640-7_18

[49] Deepe GS. *Histoplasma capsulatum* (Histoplasmosis). In: Bennet JE, Dolin R, Blaser MJ, editors. Mandell, Douglas, and Bennett's Principles and Practice of Infectious Diseases. 9th ed. Philadelphia: Elsevier; 2020. pp. 3162-3176

[50] Kwon-Chung KJ. Perfect state (Emmonsiella capsulata) of the fungus causing large-form African histoplasmosis. Mycologia. 1975;**67**(5):980-990. DOI: 10.1080/00275514.1975.12019831

[51] Kwon-Chung KJ, Weeks RJ, Larsh HW. Studies on Emmonsiella capsulata (*Histoplasma capsulatum*). II. Distribution of the two mating types in 13 endemic states of the United States. American Journal of Epidemiology. 1974;**99**(1):44-49. DOI: 10.1093/oxfordjournals.aje.a121583

[52] Rodrigues AM, Beale MA, Hagen F, Fisher MC, Terra PPD, de Hoog S, et al. The global epidemiology of emerging Histoplasma species in recent years. Studies in Mycology. 2020;**97**:100095. DOI: 10.1016/j.simyco.2020.02.001

[53] Voorhies M, Foo CK, Sil A. Experimental annotation of the human pathogen *Histoplasma capsulatum* transcribed regions using high-resolution tiling arrays. BMC Microbiology. 2011;**11**:216. DOI: 10.1186/1471-2180-11-216

[54] Mittal J, Ponce MG, Gendlina I, Nosanchuk JD. *Histoplasma capsulatum*: Mechanisms for pathogenesis. Current Topics in Microbiology and Immunology. 2019;**422**:157-191. DOI: 10.1007/82_2018_114

[55] Vincent RD, Goewert R, Goldman WE, Kobayashi GS, Lambowitz AM, Medoff G. Classification of *Histoplasma capsulatum* isolates by restriction fragment polymorphisms. Journal of Bacteriology. 1986;**165**(3):813-818. DOI: 10.1128/jb.165.3.813.1986

[56] Spitzer ED, Lasker BA, Travis SJ, Kobayashi GS, Medoff G. Use of mitochondrial and ribosomal DNA polymorphisms to classify clinical and soil isolates of *Histoplasma capsulatum*. Infection and Immunity. 1989;**57**(5):1409-1412. DOI: 10.1128/iai.57.5.1409-1412.1989

[57] Keath EJ, Kobayashi GS, Medoff G. Typing of *Histoplasma capsulatum* by restriction fragment length polymorphisms in a nuclear gene. Journal of Clinical Microbiology. 1992;**30**(8):2104-2107. DOI: 10.1128/jcm.30.8.2014-2017.1992

[58] Teixeira MM, Patané JS, Taylor ML, Gómez BL, Theodoro RC, de Hoog S, et al. Worldwide phylogenetic distributions and population dynamics of the genus Histoplasma. PLOS Neglected Tropical Diseases. 2016;**10**(6):e0004732. DOI: 10.1371/joutnal.pntd.0004732

[59] Sepúlveda VE, Márquez R, Turissini DA, Goldman WE. Matute DR,

Genome sequences reveal cryptic speciation in the human pathogen *Histoplasma capsulatum*. MBio. 2017;**8**(6):e01339-e01317. DOI: 10.1128/mBio.01339-17

[60] Davis TE, Domer JE, Li YT. Cell wall studies of *Histoplasma capsulatum* and Blastomyces dermatitis using autologous and heterologous enzymes. Infection and Immunity. 1977;**15**(3):978-987. DOI: 10.1128/iai.15.3.978-987.1977

[61] Howarth MC, Fecher RA, Deepe GS. *Histoplasma capsulatum*, lung infection and immunity. Future Microbiology. 2015;**10**:967-975. DOI: 10.2217/fmb.15.25

[62] Ray SC, Rappleye CA. Flying under the radar: *Histoplasma capsulatum* avoidance of innate immune recognition. Seminars in Cell & Developmental Biology. 2019;**89**:91-98. DOI: 10.1016/j.semcdb.2018.03.009

[63] Denham ST, Wambaugh MA, Brown JCS. How environmental fungi cause a range of clinical outcomes in susceptible hosts. Journal of Molecular Biology. 2019;**431**:2982-3009. DOI: 10.1016/j.jmb.2019.05.003

[64] Sil A. Using genomics to study the life cycle of *Histoplasma capsulatum*. In: AJP B, editor. Fungal Genomics. Berlin Heidelberg: Springer-Verlag; 2006. pp. 221-236. DOI: 10.1007/3-540-30809-1_12

[65] Okansey BK, Kosmidis C, Agyei M, Dorkenoo AM, Ayanlowo OO, Oladele RO, et al. Histoplasmosis in Africa: Current perspectives, knowledge gaps, and research priorities. PLOS Neglected Tropical Diseases. 2022;**16**(2):e0010111. DOI: 10.1371/journal.pntd.0010111

[66] de Perio MA, Benedict K, Williams SL, Niemeier-Walsh C, Green BJ, Coffey C, et al. Occupational histoplasmosis: Epidemiology and prevention measures. Journal of Fungi (Basel). 2021;**7**(7):510-522. DOI: 10.3390/jof7070510

[67] Guimarães AJ, de Cerqueira MD, Nosanchuk JD. Surface architecture of *Histoplasma capsulatum*. Frontiers in microbiology. 2011;**2**:225. DOI: 10.3389/fmicb.2011.00225

[68] Linder KA, Kauffman CA. Histoplasmosis: Epidemiology, diagnosis, and clinical manifestations. Current Fungal Infection Reports. 2019;**13**:120-128. DOI: 10.1007/s12281-019-00341-x

[69] Bahr NC, Antinori S, Wheat LJ, Sarosi GA. Histoplasmosis infections worldwide: Thinking outside of the Ohio river valley. Current Tropical Medicine Reports. 2015;**2**(2):70-80. DOI: 10.1007/s40475-015-0044-0

[70] Benedict K, Derado G, Mody RK. Histoplasmosis-associated hospitalizations in the United States, 2001-2012. Open Forum Infectious Diseases. 2016;**3**(1):ofv219. DOI: 10.1093/ofid/ofv219

[71] Azar MM, Hage CA. Clinical perspectives in the diagnosis and management of histoplasmosis. Clinics in Chest Medicine. 2017;**38**(3):403-415. DOI: 10.1016/j.ccm.2017.04.004

[72] Zerbe CS, Holland SM. Disseminated histoplasmosis in persons with interferon-γ receptor 1 deficiency. Clinical Infectious Diseases. 2005;**41**(4):38-41. DOI: 10.1086/432120

[73] Taylor ML, Pérez-Mejía A, Yamamoto-Furusho JK, Granados J. Immunologic, genetic and social human risk factors associated to histoplasmosis: Studies in the state of Guerrero. Mexico. Mycopathologia. 1997;**138**(3):137-142. DOI: 10.1023/a:1006847630347

[74] Benedict K, Thompson GR 3rd, Deresinski S, Chiller T. Mycotic infections acquired outside areas of known endemicity, United States. Emerging Infectious Disease. 2015;**21**(11):1935-1941. DOI: 10.3201/eid2111.141950

[75] Taylor ML, Reyes-Montes MDR, Estrada-BarcenasDA,Zancopé-OliveiraRM, Rodríguez-Arellanes G, Ramírez JA. Considerations about the geographic distribution of Histoplasma species. Applied and Environmental Microbiology. 2022;**88**(7):e0201021. DOI: 10.1128/aem.02010-21

[76] Ajello L. Relationship of *Histoplasma capsulatum* to avian habitats. Public Health Reports. 1964;**79**(3):266-270

[77] Deepe GS Jr. Outbreaks of histoplasmosis: The spores set sail. PLoS Pathogens. 2018;**14**(9):e1007213. DOI: 10.1371/journal.ppat.1007213

[78] Benito N, García Vázquez E, Blanco A, de Górgolas M, Gadea I, Escalonilla P, et al. Histoplasmosis diseminada en pacientes con sida. Estudio de 2 casos y revisión de la bibliografía española Disseminated histoplasmosis in AIDS patients. A study of 2 cases and review of the Spanish literature. Enfermedades Infecciosas y Microbiologia Clinica. 1998;**16**(7):316-321

[79] Gómez Londoño LF, Pérez León LC, Mcewen Ochoa JG, Zuluaga Rodriguez A, Peláez Jaramillo CA, Acevedo Ruiz JM, et al. Capacity of *Histoplasma capsulatum* to survive the composting process. Applied and Environmental Soil Science. 2019;**2019**:1-9. DOI: 10.1155/2019/5038153

[80] Carlucci JG, Halasa N, Creech CB, Dulek DE, Gómez-Duarte OG, Nelson GE, et al. Vertical transmission of histoplasmosis associated with anti-tumor necrosis factor therapy. Journal of the Pediatric Infectious Disease. 2016;**5**(2):e19-e12. DOI: 10.1093/jpids/piw001

[81] Ison MG, Nalesnik MA. An update on donor-derived disease transmission in organ transplantation. American Journal of Transplantation. 2011;**11**:1123-1130. DOI: 101111/j.1600-6143.2011.03493.x

[82] Limaye AP, Connolly PA, Sagar M, Fritsche TR, Cookson BT, Wheat LJ, et al. Transmission of *Histoplasma capsulatum* by organ transplantation. The New England Journal of Medicine. 2000;**343**(16):1163-1166. DOI: 10.1056/NEJM200010193431605

[83] Cuellar-Rodriguez J, Avery RK, Lard M, Budev M, Gordon SM, Shrestha NK, et al. Histoplasmosis in solid organ transplant recipients: 10 years of experience at a large transplant center in an endemic area. Clinical Infectious Diseases. 2009;**49**(5):710-716. DOI: 10.1086/604712

[84] Loulergue P, Bastides F, Baudouin V, Chandenier J, Mariani-Kurkdjian P, Dupont B, et al. Literature review and case histories of *Histoplasma capsulatum* var. duboisii infections in HIV-infected patients. Emerging Infectious Diseases. 2007;**13**(11):1647-1652. DOI: 10.3201/eid1311.070665

[85] Terrancle JI, Mateos RF, Solera SJ, Sánchez HV. Disseminated histoplasmosis in two brothers with AIDS. Revista Clinica Española. 2004;**204**(7):381-383. DOI: 10.1157/13063533

[86] Metzler DF, Ritter C, Culp RL. Combined effect of water purification processes on the removal of *Histoplasma capsulatum* from water. American Journal of Public Health and the Nations Health. 1956;**46**:1571-1575. DOI: 10.2105/ajph.46.12.1571

[87] Armstrong PA, Jackson BR, Haselow D, Fields V, Ireland M, Austin C, et al. Multistate epidemiology of histoplasmosis, United States, 2011-2014. Emerging Infectious Diseases. 2018;**24**(3):425-431. DOI: 10.3201/eid2403.171258

[88] Adenis AA, Aznar C, Couppié P. Histoplasmosis in HIV-infected patients: A review of new developments and remaining gaps. Current Tropical Medicine Reports. 2014;**1**(2):119-128. DOI: 10.1007/s40475-014-0017-8

[89] Wheat LJ. Histoplasmosis: A review for clinicians from non-endemic areas. Mycoses. 2006;**49**(4):274-282. DOI: 10.1111/j.1439-0507.2006.01253.x

[90] Benedict K, Mody RK. Epidemiology of histoplasmosis outbreaks, United States, 1938-2013. Emerging Infectious Diseases. 2016;**22**(3):370-378. DOI: 10.3201/eid2203.151117

[91] Queiroz-Telles F, Fahal AH, Falci DR, Caceres DH, Chiller T, Pasqualotto AC. Neglected endemic mycoses. The Lancet Infectious Diseases. 2017;**17**(11):e367-e377. DOI: 10.1016/S1473-3099(17)30306-7

[92] Kauffman CA. Histoplasmosis: A clinical and laboratory update. Clinical Microbiology Reviews. 2007;**20**(1):115-132. DOI: 10.1128/CMR.00027-06

[93] Smith DJ, Williams SL, Endemic Mycoses State Partners Group, Benedict KM, Jackson BR, Toda M. Surveillance for Coccidioidomycosis, histoplasmosis, and Blastomycosis - United States, 2019. MMWR Surveillance Summaries. 2022;**71**(7):1-14. DOI: 10.15585/mmwr.ss7107a1

[94] Ashraf N, Kubat RC, Poplin V, Adenis AA, Denning DW, Wright L, et al. Re-drawing the maps for endemic mycoses. Mycopathologia. 2020;**185**:843-865. DOI: 10.1007/s11046-020-00431-2

[95] Burden of common life-threatening fungal infections. Available from: https://gaffi.org/why/fungal-disease-frequency/ [Accessed: 2023-03-03]

[96] Centers for Disease Control (CDC). Revision of the CDC surveillance case definition for acquired immunodeficiency syndrome. Council of State and Territorial Epidemiologists; AIDS Program, Center for Infectious Diseases. MMWR Supplements. 1987;**36**(1):1S-15S

[97] Martin-Iguacel R, Kurtzhals J, Jouvion G, Nielsen SD, Llibre JM. Progressive disseminated histoplasmosis in the HIV population in Europe in the HAART era. Case report and literature review. Infection. 2014;**42**:611-620. DOI: 10.1007/s15010-014-0611-7

[98] Baker J, Setianingrum F, Wahyuningsih R, Denning DW. Mapping histoplasmosis in South East Asia - implications for diagnosis in AIDS. Emerging Microbes & Infections. 2019;**8**(1):1139-1145. DOI: 10.1080/22221751.2019.1644539

[99] McLeod DSA, Mortimer RH, Perry-Keene DA, Allworth A, Woods ML, Perry-Keene J, et al. Histoplasmosis in Australia: Report of 16 cases and literature review. Medicine (Baltimore). 2011;**90**(1):61 68. DOI: 10.1097/MD.0b013e318206e499

[100] Hepler SA, Kaufeld KA, Benedict K, Toda M, Jackson BR, Liu X, et al. Integrating public health surveillance and environmental data to model presence of Histoplasma in the United States. Epidemiology. 2022;**33**(5):654-659. DOI: 10.1097/EDE.0000000000001499

[101] Manos NE, Ferebee SH, Kerschbaum WF. Geographic variation in

the prevalence of histoplasmin sensitivity. Diseases of the Chest. 1956;**29**(6):649-668. DOI: 10.1378/chest.29.6.649

[102] Cherabie J, Mazi P, Rauseo AM, Ayres C, Larson L, Rutjanawech S, et al. Long-term mortality after Histoplasma infection in people with HIV. Journal of Fungi. 2021;**7**(5):369. DOI: 10.3390/jof7050369

[103] Brown EM, McTaggart LR, Dunn D, Pszczolko E, Tsui KG, Morris SK, et al. Epidemiology and geographic distribution of blastomycosis, histoplasmosis, and coccidioidomycosis, Ontario, Canada, 1990-2015. Emerging Infectious Diseases. 2018;**24**(7):1257-1266. DOI: 10.3201/eid2407.172063

[104] Adenis AA, Valdes A, Cropet C, McCotter OZ, Derado G, Couppie P, et al. Burden of HIV-associated histoplasmosis compared with tuberculosis in Latin America: A modeling study. The Lancet Infectious Diseases. 2018;**18**(10):1150-1159. DOI: 10.1016/S1473-3099(18)30354-2

[105] Nacher M, Leitao TS, Gómez BL, Couppié P, Adenis A, Damasceno L, et al. The fight against HIV-associated disseminated histoplasmosis in the Americas: Unfolding the different stories of four centers. Journal of Fungi. 2019;**5**(2):51. DOI: 10.3390/jof5020051

[106] Samayoa B, Roy M, Cleveland AA, Medina N, Lau-Bonilla D, Scheel CM, et al. High mortality and coinfection in a prospective cohort of human immunodeficiency virus/acquired immune deficiency syndrome patients with histoplasmosis in Guatemala. The American Journal of Tropical Medicine Hygiene. 2017;**97**(1):42-48. DOI: 10.4269/ajtmh.16-000

[107] Agudelo CA, Restrepo CA, Molina DA, Tobón AM, Kauffman CA, Murillo C, et al. Tuberculosis and histoplasmosis co-infection in AIDS patients. The American Journal of Tropical Medicine Hygiene. 2012;**87**(6):1094-1098. DOI: 10.4269/ajtmh.2012.12-0292

[108] Medina N, Alastruey-Izquierdo A, Bonilla O, Gamboa O, Mercado D, Pérez JC, et al. A rapid screening program for histoplasmosis, tuberculosis, and cryptococcosis reduces mortality in HIV patients from Guatemala. Journal of Fungi. 2021;**7**(4):268. DOI: 10.3390/jof7040268

[109] Medina N, Rodriguez-Tudela JL, Aguirre L, Salazar LR, Gamboa O, Bonilla O, et al. Incidence of histoplasmosis in a cohort of people with HIV: From estimations to reality. Microorganisms. 2021;**9**(12):2596. DOI: 10.3390/microorganisms9122596

[110] Nacher M, Adenis A, Guarmit B, Lucarelli A, Blanchet D, Demar M, et al. What is AIDS in the Amazon and the Guianas in the 90-90-90 era? PLoS One. 2020;**15**(7):e0236368. DOI: 10.1371/journal.pone.0236368

[111] Almeida MA, Almeida-Silva F, Guimarães AJ, Almeida-Paes R, Zancopé-Oliveira RM. The occurrence of histoplasmosis in Brazil: A systematic review. International Journal of Infectious Diseases. 2019;**86**:147-156. DOI: 10.1016/j.ijid.2019.07.009

[112] Brilhante RS, Fechine MA, Mesquita JR, Cordeiro RA, Rocha MFG, Monteiro AJ, et al. Histoplasmosis in HIV-positive patients in Ceará, Brazil: Clinical-laboratory aspects and in vitro antifungal susceptibility of *Histoplasma capsulatum* isolates. Transactions of the Royal Society of Tropical Medicine and Hygiene. 2012;**106**(8):484-488. DOI: 10.1016/j.trstmh.2012.05.003

[113] Oladele RO, Ayanlowo OO, Richardson MD, Denning DW.

Histoplasmosis in Africa: An emerging or a neglected disease? PLoS Neglected Tropical Disease. 2018;**12**(1):e0006046. DOI: 10.1371/journal.pntd.0006046

[114] Arlet JB, Furco-Mazzantini A, Huerre M, Neuville S, Molina JM. African histoplasmosis infection with peritoneal involvement. European Journal of Clinical Microbiololy & Infectious Diseases. 2004;**23**(4):342-344. DOI: 10.1007/s10096-003-1089-x

[115] Kneale M, Bartholomew JS, Davies E, Denning DW. Global access to antifungal therapy and its variable cost. The Journal of Antimicrobial Chemotherapy. 2016;**71**(12):3599-3606. DOI: 10.1093/jac/dkw325

[116] Pan B, Chen M, Pan W, Liao W. Histoplasmosis: A new endemic fungal infection in China? Review and analysis of cases. Mycoses. 2013;**56**(3):212-221. DOI: 10.1111/myc.12029

[117] Zhao B, Xia X, Yin J, Zhang X, Wu E, Shi Y, et al. Epidemiological investigation of *Histoplasma capsulatum* infection in China. Chinese Medical Journal (English). 2001;**114**(7):743-746

[118] Wen FQ, Sun YD, Watanabe K, Yoshida MJ, JNS W, Baum GL. Prevalence of histoplasmin sensitivity in healthy adults and tuberculosis patients in Southwest China. Journal of Medical and Veterinary Mycology. 1996;**34**(3):171-174. DOI: 10.1080/02681219680000281

[119] Taylor RL, Duangmani C, Charoenvit Y. The geographic distribution of histoplasmin sensitivity in Thailand. The American Journal of Tropical Medicine and Hygiene. 1968;**17**(4):579-583. DOI: 10.4269/ajtmh.1968.17.579

[120] Norkaew T, Ohno H, Sriburee P, Tanabe K, Tharavichitkul P, Takarn P, et al. Detection of environmental sources of *Histoplasma capsulatum* in Chiang Mai, Thailand, by nested PCR. Mycopathologia. 2013;**176**(5-6):395-402. DOI: 10.1007/s11046-013-9701-9

[121] Tucker HA, Kvisselgaard N. Histoplasmin and tuberculin sensitivity in Burma; study of tests on 3,558 subjects. Bulletin World Health Organization. 1952;**7**(2):188-200

[122] Sanyal M, Thammayya A. *Histoplasma capsulatum* in the soil of Gangetic plain in India. The Indian Journal of Medical Research. 1975;**63**(7):1020-1028

[123] Goswami RP, Pramanik N, Banerjee D, Raza MM, Guha SK, Maiti PK. Histoplasmosis in eastern India: The tip of the iceberg? Transactions of the Royal Society of Tropical Medicine and Hygiene. 1999;**93**(5):540-542. DOI: 10.1016/S0035-9203(99)90374-7

[124] Gupta A, Ghosh A, Singh G, Xess I. A twenty-first-century perspective of disseminated histoplasmosis in India: Literature review and retrospective analysis of published and unpublished cases at a tertiary care hospital in North India. Mycopathologia. 2017;**182**(11-12):1077-1093. DOI: 10.1007/s11046-017-0191-z

[125] Randhawa HS, Khan ZU. Histoplasmosis in India: Current status. The Indian Journal Chest Diseases and Allied Sciences. 1994;**36**(4):193, 213

[126] Kikuchi K, Sugita T, Makimura K, Urata K, Someya T, Sasaki T, et al. Is *Histoplasma capsulatum* a native inhabitant of Japan? Microbiology and Immunology. 2008;**52**:455-459. DOI: 10.1111/j.1348-0421.2008.00052.x

[127] Sabino R, Verissímo C, Brandão J, Martins C, Alves D, Pais C, et al. Serious

fungal infections in Portugal. European Journal of Clinical Microbiology & Infectious Diseases. 2017;**36**(7):1345-1352. DOI: 10.1007/s10096-017-2930-y

[128] Ashbee HR, Evans EG, Viviani MA, Dupont B, Chryssanthou E, Surmont I, et al. Histoplasmosis in Europe: Report on an epidemiological survey from the European Confederation of Medical Mycology Working Group. Medical Mycology. 2008;**46**(1):57-65. DOI: 10.1080/13693780701591481

[129] Sotgiu G, Mazzoni A, Mantovani A, Ajello L, Palmer J. *Histoplasma capsulatum*: Occurrence in soil from the Emilia-Romagna region of Italy. Science. 1965;**147**(3658):624. DOI: 10.1126/science.147.3658.624

[130] Mantovani A, Mazzoni A, Ajello L. Histoplasmosis in Italy. I. Isolation of *Histoplasma capsulatum* from dogs in the province of Bologna. Sabouraudia. 1968;**6**(2):163-164. DOI: 10.1080/00362176885190291

[131] Poveda F, García-Alegría J, de las Nieves MA, Villar E, Montiel N, del Arco A. Disseminated histoplasmosis successfully treated with liposomal amphotericin B following azathioprine therapy in a patient from a nonendemic area. European Journal of Clinical Microbiology & Infectious Diseases. 1998;**17**(5):357-359. DOI: 10.1007/BF01709461

[132] Antinori S, Giacomelli A, Corbellino M, Torre A, Schiuma M, Casalini G, et al. Histoplasmosis diagnosed in Europe and Israel: A case report and systematic review of the literature from 2005 to 2020. Journal of Fungi (Basel). 2021;**7**(6):481-502. DOI: 10.3390/jof7060481

[133] Goodwin RA, Lloyd JE, Des Prez RM. Histoplasmosis in normal hosts. Medicine (Baltimore). 1981;**60**(4):231-266. DOI: 10.1097/00005792-198107000-00001

[134] Shen Q, Rappleye CA. Living within the macrophage: Dimorphic fungal pathogen intracellular metabolism. Frontiers in Cellular and Infection Microbiology. 2020;**10**:592259. DOI: 10.3389/fcimb.2020.592259

[135] Newman SL, Gootee L, Bullock WE. Inhibition of intracellular growth of *Histoplasma capsulatum* yeast cells by cytokine-activated human monocytes and macrophages. Infection and immunity. 1991;**59**(2):737-741. DOI: 10.1128/iai.59.2.737-741.1991

[136] Fojtasek MF, Sherman MR, Garringer T, Blair R, Wheat LJ, Schnizlein-Bick CT. Local immunity in lung-associated lymph nodes in a murine model of pulmonary histoplasmosis. Infection and Immunity. 1993;**61**(11):4607-4614. DOI: 10.1128/iai.61.11.4607-4614.1993

[137] Guimarães AJ, Nosanchuk JD, Zancopé-Oliveira RM. Diagnosis of histoplasmosis. Brazilian Journal of Microbiology. 2006;**37**:1-13. DOI: 10.1590/s1517-83822006000100001

[138] Newman SL, Gootee L, Gabay JE. Human neutrophil-mediated fungistasis against *Histoplasma capsulatum*. Localization of fungistatic activity to the azurophil granules. Journal of Clinical Investigation. 1993;**92**(2):624-631. DOI: 10.1172/jci116630

[139] Lin JS, Huang JH, Hung LY, Wu SY, Wu-Hsieh BA. Distinct roles of complement receptor 3, Dectin-1, and sialic acids in murine macrophage interaction with Histoplasma yeast. Journal of Leukocyte Biology. 2010;**88**:95-106. DOI: 10.1189/jlb.1109717

[140] Lin JS, Yang CW, Wang DW, Wu-Hsieh BA. Dendritic cells cross-present exogenous fungal antigens to stimulate a protective CD8 T cell response in infection by *Histoplasma capsulatum*. Journal of Immunology. 2005;**174**:6282-6291. DOI: 10.4049/jimmunol.174.10.6282

[141] Nosanchuk JD, Gacser A. *Histoplasma capsulatum* at the host-pathogen interface. Microbes and Infection. 2008;**10**:973-977. DOI: 10.1016/j.micinf.2008.07.011]

[142] Roth MT, Zamith-Miranda D, Nosanchuk JD. Immunization strategies for the control of histoplasmosis. Current Tropical Medicine Reports. 2019;**6**(2):35-41. DOI: 10.1007/s40475-019-00172-3

[143] Almeida PCS, Roque BS, Felice AG, Jaiswal AK, Tiwari S, Azevedo V, et al. Comparative genomics of *Histoplasma capsulatum* and prediction of new vaccines and drug targets. Journal of Fungi. 2023;**9**:193. DOI: 10.3390/jof9020193

[144] McKinsey DS, Wheat LJ, Cloud GA, Pierce M, Black JR, Bamberger DM, et al. Itraconazole prophylaxis for fungal infections in patients with advanced human immunodeficiency virus infection: Randomized, placebo-controlled, double-blind study. National Institute of Allergy and Infectious Diseases mycoses study group. Clinical Infectious Diseases. 1999;**28**(5):1049-1056. DOI: 10.1085/514744

[145] Miller R, Assi M. Endemic fungal infections in solid organ transplantation. American Journal of Transplantation. 2013;**13**:25-261. DOI: 10.1111/ajt.12117

[146] Wallis RS, Broder M, Wong J, Lee A, Hoq L. Reactivation of latent granulomatous infections by infliximab. Clinical Infectious Diseases. 2005;**41**(3):194-198. DOI: 10.1086/429996

Chapter 3

Epidemiology and Knowledge Gap of Histoplasmosis in Africa

Israel Kiiza Njovu, Pauline Petra Nalumaga, Kennedy Kassaza, Lucas Ampaire, Edwin Nuwagira, Joel Bazira and Herbert Itabangi

Abstract

A dimorphic fungus called *Histoplasma capsulatum* is the cause of the granulomatous disease known as histoplasmosis. *Histoplasma capsulatum var. capsulatum* (Hcc) and *Histoplasma capsulatum var. duboisii* (Hcd), 2 variants of this fungus can infect humans and cause, classical or American histoplasmosis and African histoplasmosis, respectively. To improve the knowledge of health professionals, awareness of most fungal diseases, such as histoplasmosis, has been increased in Africa. In this review, we provide an overview of the current status of histoplasmosis in Africa, identify information gaps, and suggest targets for further study. The histoplasmosis literature in medical mycology textbooks and published articles from Google Scholar on histoplasmosis in Africa and the rest of the world were searched and reviewed. There was no restriction on the year of publications Conclusions were drawn from this review. Whereas the Western world has advanced technologies to diagnose histoplasmosis, this is not the case in Africa. Pulmonary histoplasmosis is therefore usually misdiagnosed as pulmonary tuberculosis because it has a similar clinical presentation. Due to a lack of knowledge and diagnostic tools, most national health systems in Africa are unable to correctly diagnose histoplasmosis, leading to misdiagnosis of the disease despite the fact that the continent has a sizable population of HIV/AIDS patients who are susceptible to contracting the illness. Under-recognition and under-diagnosis remain key issues caused by the lack of competent workers and diagnostic facilities. Therefore, this issue must be addressed by coordinated efforts. Also, it is crucial for doctors practicing outside of endemic areas to understand this illness' symptoms and treatment options. This is especially significant in light of African migration patterns.

Keywords: histoplasmosis, epidemiology, knowledge gap, misdiagnosis, tuberculosis

1. Introduction

One of the endemic mycoses is histoplasmosis. A fungal disease is caused by dimorphic fungi, that typically grow as yeasts at body temperature but exist in the environment as mycelial forms in the soil. Other endemic mycoses are blastomycosis, coccidioidomycosis, paracoccidioidomycosis, sporotrichosis, and penicilliosis, and they are all restricted to particular geographical areas and epidemiological contexts

[1]. Histoplasmosis often spreads through airborne conidia inhalation, similar to other endemic mycoses, yet in some instances, the fungus is inoculated through the skin. Clinically, histoplasmosis presentation largely dependent on the host's immune status. For immunocompetent persons, primary infection may be symptomatic and may resolve on its own. However, initial infection typically escalates to widespread disease in patients with weakened host defense, such as transplant recipients taking immunosuppressive medication and HIV patients. *Histoplasma capsulatum* has the ability to develop into a mold in soil or culture at temperatures below 30°C, and a yeast-like fungus in living tissue at 37°C is due to its dimorphism characteristic. There are three varieties of *Histoplasma capsulatum* depending on the clinical disease: *Histoplasma capsulatum* var. *capsulatum* (Hcc), the cause of Classical histoplasmosis, also known as the American histoplasmosis; *Histoplasma capsulatum* var. *duboisii* (Hcd) also known as the African type of histoplamosis that causes African histoplasmosis and *Histoplasma capsulatum* var. *farciminosum* causes lymphangitis among equines. Soil rich in chicken, starling, and bat droppings has been used to create fungal environmental isolations.

This chapter investigates the epidemiology of the histoplasmosis pandemic in Africa as well as the knowledge gap among healthcare professionals.

2. Epidemiology

Histoplasmosis is a disease that affects people all over the world, but it is especially prevalent in North and Central America and South America along the valleys of the Ohio and Mississippi Rivers. It has been identified in Madagascar, West Africa, South Africa, Eastern and Central Africa, and Africa. Additionally, isolated cases from the Mediterranean Basin and Southeast Asia have been documented [2–5]. Uganda, Nigeria, the Democratic Republic of the Congo, and Senegal are the countries where African histoplasmosis disease has been most frequently documented, as Hcd only occurs on the continent of Africa. African histoplasmosis accounted for 61% of the 470 histoplasmosis cases that were documented in Africa from 1952 to 2017 [3]. Central and western Africa accounted for 87% of all cases of histoplasmosis in Africa. Eastern and Southern Africa have recorded fewer occurrences than other continents. The bulk of histoplasmosis cases found in southern Africa are caused by Hcc, whereas Hcd is more common in the west, central Africa, and 4Madagascar [6]. The majority (n = 119) of the 150 cases that were reported from Southern Africa were brought on by *H. capsulatum var. capsulatum* (Hcc), and neither Hcd nor Hcc had any case reports from Northern Africa [6]. It's important to remember that, unlike Hcd, which is only found in Africa, Hcc is more prevalent in North and South America, even if it can also be found in Europe, Asia, and other parts of the world.

The predominance of Hcd in Africa has been confirmed by the 400 cases of African histoplasmosis alone that have been reported from 32 African nations in 2020, either as case reports or as case series [7]. In the Democratic Republic of the Congo and Togo, studies conducted during the previous six and fifteen years, respectively, identified 17 and 36 cases [8, 9].

Surveys of Histoplasma skin sensitivity remain crucial for identifying endemic regions or preclinical histoplasmosis. However, a survey conducted in Nigeria, revealed a 4% Histoplasma skin-positive rate [10]. Histoplasmosis is an unknown public health concern in Africa that is mistakenly diagnosed for tuberculosis, as evidenced by the detection of *H. capsulatum* in 13% of HIV-infected individuals in Cameroonian research [11]. It's vital to avoid undervaluing the diagnosis of disseminated histoplasmosis (HD) in HIV-infected people due to the endemicity of tuberculosis, the main HIV-defining disease in Africa.

According to various case studies, 2:1 more men than women contract histoplasmosis [8]. Cases have been documented among people between 13 months and 70 years, but all age groups may be affected [12]. Histoplasmosis, particularly classical histoplasmosis, frequently co-occurs with TB and HIV and is expected to be a major health burden in sub-Saharan Africa. However, there appears to be little correlation between HIV and African histoplasmosis [13]. Epizootic histoplasmosis can affect nonhuman primates, including dogs, cats, horses, baboons, and dogs. In Ethiopia, an African nation, equine histoplasmosis has been extensively reported [14]. A recent case of histoplasmosis associated with Hcd in a baboon in America has been related to the import of baboons from Senegal [15]. Still, there is lack of evidence for either human-to-human or animal-to-animal transmission.

3. Knowledge gap

The prevalence of histoplasmosis in Africa is unclear. Consequently, the disease's burden is underestimated. The largest rate of HIV infection, which increases the risk of histoplasmosis, is found in Africa [16]. Whereas the Western world has advanced technologies to diagnose histoplasmosis, it's not the same case in Africa. Thus, there is a general knowledge gap among health workers in Africa to diagnose histoplasmosis. Pulmonary histoplasmosis could be mostly misdiagnosed as pulmonary tuberculosis since it presents with similar clinical presentations. On the same note, histoplasmosis skin test surveys done in Africa indicated a 0–35% positive rate which proves there is an existing unknown burden of histoplasmosis [3]. As a result of clinical signs that are similar to TB, histoplasmosis is frequently mistaken as TB. Because histoplasmosis and tuberculosis (TB) present clinically similarly, some misdiagnoses may occur due to a lack of diagnostic resources. Both pulmonary TB and chronic pulmonary histoplasmosis have similar signs and symptoms, such as malaise, fever, lethargy, cough, and sputum production. However, sputum production, weight loss, and night sweats are less common in histoplasmosis patients than in TB. Chronic pulmonary histoplasmosis frequently progresses to pulmonary insufficiency at some point. Histoplasmosis rarely kills if untreated in immune-competent people, unlike TB in an advanced stage [1].

Studies comparing TB with histoplasmosis in the presence of HIV infection found that while the two diseases have many traits, with the majority of publications concentrating on disseminated Hcc infection, however, there are also important and substantial differences between the two diseases [11]. Disseminated histoplasmosis is common in the HIV/AIDS context, typically with lung involvement, but other clinical signs are more apparent, most prominently diarrhea and other gastrointestinal symptoms, skin lesions, and pancytopenia that vary by region. In 8–15% of cases, there has been evidence of co-infection with histoplasmosis. Reticulonodular lesions, many pulmonary nodules, hilar and mediastinal adenopathy, and advancing fibrosis are further characteristics.

Patients that are misdiagnosed with tuberculosis instead of histoplasmosis due to clinical similarities [17, 18] frequently receive presumptive anti-tuberculosis therapy, even when tuberculosis has not been diagnosed. The patients eventually pass away from what is most likely disseminated histoplasmosis (DH), and postmortem tissue samples may ultimately reveal the fungus infection [19]. Despite not being on the World Health Organization's official list, Hcd histoplasmosis is regarded as a neglected tropical illness. Since the first report in 1952, about only 400 Hcd cases have been documented;

nevertheless, due to the small number of case series, the epidemiologic and clinical traits as well as the best therapeutic therapy are still unknown [7]. As previously mentioned, there are few options for laboratory diagnosis in low-income countries, and 55% of cases may only be determined through direct inspection or histological study of clinical specimen(s). As a result, several diagnoses are in doubt [7].

According to studies, the frequency of Hcd infection is likely underestimated since cases are frequently ignored, particularly in developing countries with limited incomes. As a result of the disease's very pleiomorphic clinical presentation, it ought to be considered quite often. The prevalence of HIV coinfection (20% of patients) significantly alters this clinical picture. Most diagnoses are made through direct examination, which calls for specialized laboratory supplies and microscopist abilities that aren't usually available in Africa.

There is an urgent need for more precise and user-friendly diagnostic tools to confirm diagnoses and distinguish between Hcd and Hcc disorders, both of which are prevalent on the African continent. When seen under a direct microscope, Histoplasma var. duboisii typically stands out from Hcc due to the abundance of big yeasts it displays.

4. Diagnosis

Histoplasmosis differential diagnosis usually begins with clinical presentation in a patient; however, these clinical signs and symptoms are not always specific because they are similar to those of other diseases like pulmonary tuberculosis, mistaking it for classical histoplasmosis. Unlike classical histoplasmosis which normally affects the lungs and at dissemination, affects the central nervous system (brain and the spinal cord); Osteoarticular, ganglionic, and very infrequently pulmonary sites are affected by African histoplasmosis [8, 20]. Rare incidences of urogenital skin injury often involve secondary skin invasions in people with widespread cases [21, 22]. African histoplasmosis also presents clinically as a "localized skin, bone, lymph node infections or as disseminated with multiple cutaneous lesions present all over the body, subcutaneous abscesses, enlarged lymph nodes, liver and spleen, and visceral organ enlargement [20, 23, 24]. Cutaneous manifestations are clearly isolated, and sometimes present with nodules, papules, or ulcers [20, 25]. Most frequent symptoms of Hcd include lesions mainly on the limbs, trunk, and face; osteoarticular infections in the spine, thorax, and bones of the upper and lower limbs; superficial and deep-seated lymphadenopathies. Rarely does Hcd cause infection in the Lungs, Adrenal glands, and nasal or buccal cavity, gastrointestinal tract (gastric or duodenal lesions), peritoneal cavity [7]. In general, Hcd manifestation is different from classical histoplasmosis, usually affecting bones and the skin and infrequently the lungs [4], and it has been observed in HIV infections less frequently than Hcc [26–29]. Microscopy and culture are the only readily available diagnostic tools in Africa; serological, immunological, radiological, and molecular methods are still lacking, and are therefore unable to be used to diagnose histoplasmosis (for example, by detecting the *H. capsulatum* circulating antigen in bodily fluids using an enzyme immunoassay methods) [30].

Histoplasmosis is diagnosed with microscopic histopathologic investigations of bone marrow aspirate or biopsy material, bronchoalveolar lavage fluid or lung biopsy material, sputum, urine, white blood cells in peripheral blood, and skin lesions [31–35]. Microscopically, Hcd is identified as an ovoid budding yeast with thick cell walls, bigger (6–12 m in diameter), and intracellular fat droplets [36]. On the histology of a tissue specimen, Hcc however, shows up as 2–4um narrow-based budding yeast [36]. Other yeasts can be distinguished from Histoplasma yeasts by their dominant cellular location (intracellular for *H. capsulatum* and extracellular for *C. glabrata*), size and form variation (uniform versus heterogeneous), and histopathologic response (granulomatous versus suppurative). It is possible to distinguish between these infections by using particular histochemical stains, such as periodic acid-Schiff, Gomori methenamine silver, hematoxylin and eosin, and Giemsa [36]. A conclusive diagnosis of invasive infection is made by histopathologic analysis of the bone marrow [37]. These microscopic examinations are important in alerting the laboratory about a suspectible pathogen [38]. However, due to the *H. capsulatum* yeasts similar structure to other yeasts such as *Candida glabrata*, *Penicillium marneffei, Pneumocystis (carinii) jeroveci, Toxoplasma gondii, Leishmania donovani and Cryptococcus neoformans* many diagnostic techniques lack sensitivity and specificity which can lead to misidiagnosis [39–41].

Having access to a level 3 biosafety facility is necessary for culture since it poses a risk to laboratory staff and is not commonly found in African healthcare settings [17]. The culture, isolation, and confirmation of H. capsulatum from clinical and biological materials on selective media, such as Sabouraud agar, and incubation at 25°C for 6 to 12 weeks still serve as the basis for the final diagnosis. When incubated at 35–37°C, *H. capsulatum* molds are microscopically made up of hyaline septated hyphae with micro and tuberculate. Although the rate of conversion is modest and makes the procedure unusable as a diagnostic tool, it has been used to demonstrate that *H. capsulatum* is dimorphic. After conversion, smooth white to brown yeast colonies are seen and on microscopic examination, small round narrow budding yeasts are observed [38]. Gram-stained *H. capsulatum* exhibits poor staining compared to yeast cells from Candida and Cryptococcus, which are primarily extracellular macroconidia. Through culturing on enriched media like blood agar or Brain-Heart Infusion Agar (BHI) containing cysteine, *H. caspulatum* can be converted from to yeast phase. The majority of patients with an asymptomatic or moderate form of histoplasmosis have negative cultures since culture diagnosis is 100% specific but its sensitivity relies on the number of fungi present [41]. The most recent BACTEC type [42] is more successful than both lysis centrifugation and traditional biphasic blood systems [43, 44]. However, lysis centrifugation has more sensitivity than conventional and Bactec MYCO/F Lytic blood cultures for the recovery of *H. capsulatum* [45].

There are currently no molecular assays for *H. capsulatum* accepted by the FDA that are directly applicable to clinical specimens; however, laboratory-developed PCR assays using a range of target genes have been developed and show more sensitivity than cultures, such as between 59 and 100% [46] and 33 and 87% [47–49]. There is no recorded molecular method that has been used to detect histoplasmosis in Africa. The general lack of expertise in Africa to skillfully diagnose histoplasmosis makes it difficult to accurately diagnose histoplasmosis. Academic tertiary institutions provide theoretical knowledge but cannot provide practical high-end standard methods for diagnosing histoplasmosis. In situations where there is a minimal fungal burden, such as in asymptomatic or chronic pulmonary histoplasmosis, serology tests for anti-Histoplasma antibodies are incredibly helpful [1, 17]. Immunocompromised HIV-infected patients have lower sensitivity to antibody detection by immuno-diffusion or complement fixation than immunocompetent patients [50, 51]. Anti-H and anti-M antibody detection is the main focus of serologic diagnosis. Histoplasmin (HMIN) can be used to identify such antibodies. The antigenic extract of H. capsulatum mycelial culture is identified as HMIN. Centrifugation at 1050 × g for 10 min is used to remove the cells, and the supernatant is then filtered through a 0.45 m membrane, concentrated and dialyzed using phosphate-buffered saline (PBS) [52–57]. The M antigen is a catalase [58, 59] while the H antigen is a β-glucosidase [55]. Antibodies against the M and H antigens can be especially helpful in diagnosis due to their increased specificity to *H. capsulatum* [60–62]. Precipitating antibodies (H and M precipitin lines or bands) are qualitatively measured by the immunodiffusion (ID) test [63, 64]. Due to a noted rise in false-negative results, these approaches should not be utilized in patients with the disseminated type of histoplasmosis. As Histoplasma-like antigens are present in patients with other prevalent pathogens such TB, lymphoma, sarcoidosis, and other fungal diseases [65], serologic cross-reactions may happen. Western blot test strips have shown high sensitivity and specificity rates [66]. However, Miravista Histoplasma antibody enzyme immunoassay (EIA) has proved to be more sensitive than other antibody assays, detecting both immunoglobulin G (IgG) and IgM antibodies, and complements antigen detection [67]. Thus becoming the best method to diagnose acute pulmonary histoplasmosis by combining antigen and EIA antibody tests. The invention of Histoplasma antigen testing has greatly aided in the diagnosis of disseminated histoplasmosis. A variety of EIA techniques have been used to find Hcc circulating antigens. Patients with immunosuppressed are more sensitive to disseminated histoplasmosis antigen testing in blood or urine, and individuals with a more severe illness have greater titers [68, 69]. The extent of the disease is proportional to the antigen level [70]. However, one of the gold standards for identifying histoplasmosis in immunocompromised patients remains Histoplasma antigen testing. The Histoplasma antigen does not interact with *C. neoformans* [71, 72]. Serology was only identified as being used to make a diagnosis in five African countries (Tanzania, Benin, South Africa, Egypt, and Uganda), and in three of those instances, the samples were processed in Western countries. Histology and culture were used to diagnose most reported cases from Africa [3].

5. Treatment

The preferred medications for treating histoplasmosis are intravenous amphotericin B and itraconazole. However, these medications are extremely expensive and scarcely available in Africa. Therefore, the antifungal medications used to treat Hcd and Hcc infection, primarily intravenous amphotericin B and itraconazole, must be made available at a lower cost [3]. Histoplasmosis laboratory diagnosis typically takes a long turnaround time, which raises the risk of the disease progressing.

Whether or not a patient exhibits notable symptoms, doctors have two alternatives for starting treatment for those with a high probability of having histoplasmosis: intravenous (IV) amphotericin B or oral itraconazole [30]. Even though it is frequently fungicidal and has proven beneficial in terms of survival, amphotericin B is nephrotoxic [73]. Liposomal amphotericin is superior to traditional amphotericin B for treating disseminated histoplasmosis, especially in AIDS patients with compromised immune systems [73]. For the majority of isolates of *H. capsulatum*, itraconazole is similarly fungicidal; however, oral capsules are not always well absorbed in advanced AIDS patients, and it is linked to numerous medication interactions, including rifampicin for situations when TB is present. Itraconazole is a good alternative for subacute disseminated infection, but amphotericin B is preferred for the initial treatment of AIDS-related disseminated histoplasmosis [30]. Amphotericin B is unlicensed and unavailable in several African nations, which is concerning yet when available, the price could be exorbitant [74]. Amphotericin B liposomal is extremely expensive and unavailable throughout most of Africa. Despite being accessible in the most of African nations, itraconazole is excessively expensive [74].

6. Conclusion

Most of Africa's health national health systems are incapacitated to diagnose histoplasmosis due to a lack of expertise and diagnostic technologies, thus causing miss diagnosis of the same disease. However, the continent also includes a sizable population of HIV/AIDS patients at risk of contracting the illness. Due to a shortage of trained persons and facilities to perform this diagnosis, it is inevitable to misdiagnose histoplasmosis. Coordinated efforts must be undertaken to address this. In addition, medical professionals practicing outside of endemic areas need to understand this disease and how to treat it. Considering the migration patterns of African migrants, this is of great importance [75].

Acknowledgements

I acknowledge EDCTP, European Union, MUST and MeMoF project for the support and funding provided for this work.

Author details

Israel Kiiza Njovu[1*], Pauline Petra Nalumaga[1], Kennedy Kassaza[2], Lucas Ampaire[3], Edwin Nuwagira[4], Joel Bazira[2] and Herbert Itabangi[5]

1 Faculty of Medicine, Department of Microbiology, Mycology Unit, Mbarara University of Science and Technology, Mbarara, Uganda

2 Faculty of Medicine, Department of Microbiology, Mbarara University of Science and Technology, Mbarara, Uganda

3 Faculty of Medicine, Department of Medical Laboratory Science, Mbarara University of Science and Technology, Mbarara, Uganda

4 Faculty of Medicine, Department of Internal Medicine, Mbarara University of Science and Technology, Mbarara, Uganda

5 Faculty of Health Sciences, Department of Microbiology and Immunology, Busitema University, Mbale, Uganda

*Address all correspondence to: israelkin25@gmail.com

References

[1] Anaissie EJ, McGinnis MR, Pfaller MA. Clinical Mycology E-Book. Annals of Internal Medicine. Philadelphia: Elsevier Health Sciences; 2009

[2] Ekeng BE, Oladele RO, Emanghe UE, Ochang EA, Mirabeau TY. Prevalence of histoplasmosis and molecular characterization of histoplasma species in patients with presumptive pulmonary tuberculosis in Calabar, Nigeria. Open Forum Infectious Diseases. Arlington, Virginia: Infectios Diseases Society of America; 2022

[3] Oladele RO, Ayanlowo OO, Richardson MD, Denning DW. Histoplasmosis in Africa: An emerging or a neglected disease? PLoS Neglected Tropical Diseases. 2018;**12**(1):e0006046

[4] Kuate MPN, Nyasa R, Mandengue C, Tendongfor N, Bongomin F, Denning DW. Screening for acute disseminated histoplasmosis in HIV disease using urinary antigen detection enzyme immunoassay: A pilot study in Cameroon. Journal of Microbiological Methods. 2021;**185**:106226

[5] Oladele R, Osaigbovo I, Akanmu A, Adekanmbi O, Ekeng B, Mohammed Y, et al. Ascertaining the current prevalence of histoplasmosis in Nigeria's advanced HIV disease population. Emerging Infectious Diseases. 2022;**28**:2261-2269

[6] Bongomin F, Ekeng BE, Kibone W, Nsenga L, Olum R, Itam-Eyo A, et al. Invasive fungal diseases in Africa: A critical literature review. Journal of Fungi. 2022;**8**(12):1236

[7] Develoux M, Amona F, Hennequin C. Histoplasmosis caused by Histoplasma capsulatum var. duboisii: A comprehensive review of cases from 1993 to 2019. Clinical Infectious Diseases. 2021;**73**(3):e543-e5e9

[8] Darré T, Saka B, Mouhari-Touré A, Dorkenoo AM, Amégbor K, Pitche VP, et al. Histoplasmosis by Histoplasma capsulatum var. duboisii observed at the laboratory of pathological anatomy of Lomé in Togo. Journal of Pathogens. 2017;**2017**:2

[9] Pakasa N, Biber A, Nsiangana S, Imposo D, Sumaili E, Muhindo H, et al. African histoplasmosis in HIV-negative patients, Kimpese, Democratic Republic of the Congo. Emerging Infectious Diseases. 2018;**24**(11):2068

[10] Oladele RO, Toriello C, Ogunsola FT, Ayanlowo OO, Foden P, Fayemiwo AS, et al. Prior subclinical histoplasmosis revealed in Nigeria using histoplasmin skin testing. PLoS One. 2018;**13**(5):e0196224

[11] Mandengue CE, Ngandjio A, Atangana PJ. Histoplasmosis in HIV-infected persons, Yaoundé, Cameroon. Emerging Infectious Diseases. 2015;**21**(11):2094

[12] Ashbee H, Evans E, Viviani M, Dupont B, Chryssanthou E, Surmont I, et al. Histoplasmosis in Europe: Report on an epidemiological survey from the European Confederation of Medical Mycology Working Group. Medical Mycology. 2008;**46**(1):57-65

[13] Lucas AO. Cutaneous manifestations of African histoplasmosis. British Journal of Dermatology. 1970;**82**(5):435-447

[14] Paugam A, de Pécoulas P, Bourée P. African young girl with sores of the elbow, cold abcesses and Molluscum-like cutaneous lesions. Lett Infect. 2014;**7**(4):126-129

[15] Hensel M, Hoffmann AR, Gonzales M, Owston M, Dick E Jr. Phylogenetic analysis of Histoplasma capsulatum var duboisii in baboons from archived formalin-fixed, paraffin embedded tissues. Medical Mycology. 2019;**57**(2):256-259

[16] De Cock KM, Mbori-Ngacha D, Marum E. Shadow on the continent: Public health and HIV/AIDS in Africa in the 21st century. The Lancet. 2002;**360**(9326):67-72

[17] Couppié P, Aznar C, Carme B, Nacher M. American histoplasmosis in developing countries with a special focus on patients with HIV: Diagnosis, treatment, and prognosis. Current Opinion in Infectious Diseases. 2006;**19**(5):443-449

[18] Jeong HW, Sohn J-W, Kim MJ, Choi JW, Kim CH, Choi S-H, et al. Disseminated histoplasmosis and tuberculosis in a patient with HIV infection. Yonsei Medical Journal. 2007;**48**(3):531-534

[19] Mandengue C, Lindou J, Mandeng N, Takuefou B, Nouedoui C, Atangana P, et al. Fatal miliary tuberculosis in an HIV-infected Cameroon woman: Disseminated histoplasmosis due to Histoplasma capsulatum capsulatum. Medecine Tropicale: Revue du Corps de Sante Colonial. 2011;**71**(6):615-617

[20] Darré T, Kpatcha M, Djiwa T, Sewa E, Dorkenoo AM, Kouyaté M, et al. African histoplasmosis of the penis. Oxford Medical Case Reports. 2020;**2020**(6):omaa043

[21] Cipriano A, Neves-Maia J, Lopes V, Fleming C, Ferreira M, Bathay J. African histoplasmosis in a Guinea Bissau patient with HIV-2: Case report and review. Journal de mycologie médicale. 2020;**30**(1):100904

[22] Pasqualotto AC, Oliveira FM, Severo LC. Histoplasma capsulatum recovery from the urine and a short review of genitourinary histoplasmosis. Mycopathologia. 2009;**167**:315-323

[23] Paixão M, Miot HA, Avancini J, Belda JW. Primary cutaneous histoplasmosis developed in the penis of an immunocompetent patient. Anais Brasileiros de Dermatologia. 2015;**90**:255-257

[24] Chaurasia D, Agrawal R, Misra V, Bhargava A. Penoscrotal histoplasmosis following bladder carcinoma. International Journal of Urology. 2007;**14**(6):571-572

[25] Sachdev R, Goel RK, Malviya S, Goel S, Gajendra S. Scrotal histoplasmosis masquerading as Fournier's gangrene. International Journal of Surgical Pathology. 2017;**25**(6):509-510

[26] Deepe GS Jr. Histoplasma Capsulatum (Histoplasmosis). Mandell, Douglas, and Bennett's Principles and Practice of Infectious Diseases. Amsterdam, Netherlands: Elsevier; 2015. pp. 2949-2962 e1

[27] Carme B, Ngolet A, Ebikili B, Ngaporo AI. Is African histoplasmosis an opportunistic fungal infection in AIDS? Transactions of the Royal Society of Tropical Medicine and Hygiene. Mar-Apr 1990;**84**(2):293. DOI: 10.1016/0035-9203(90)90292-m. PMID: 2389325

[28] Chandenier J, Goma D, Moyen G, Samba-Lefèbvre M-C, Nzingoula S, Mbitsi A, et al. African histoplasmosis, Histoplasma capsulatum var. duboisii: Relationship with Aids in recent Congolese cases. Cahiers d'études et de recherches francophones/Santé. 1995;**5**(4):227-234

[29] Antinori S, Magni C, Nebuloni M, Parravicini C, Corbellino M, Sollima S, et al. Histoplasmosis among human immunodeficiency virus-infected

people in Europe: Report of 4 cases and review of the literature. Medicine. 2006;**85**(1):22-36

[30] Adenis AA, Aznar C, Couppié P. Histoplasmosis in HIV-infected patients: A review of new developments and remaining gaps. Current Tropical Medicine Reports. 2014;**1**:119-128

[31] Atkinson G, Randall E. The diagnosis of fungal infections of the respiratory tract. Annals of Clinical & Laboratory Science. 1973;**3**(3):194-200

[32] Baughman RP, Kim CK, Bullock WE. Comparative diagnostic efficacy of bronchoalveolar lavage, transbronchial biopsy, and open-lung biopsy in experimental pulmonary histoplasmosis. The Journal of Infectious Diseases. 1986;**153**(2):376-377

[33] Davis O, Wolff A. Pathologic diagnosis: Histoplasmosis of the tonsil. Archives of Otolaryngology (Chicago, Ill: 1960). 1985;**111**(8):558-560

[34] Moffit GW, Morgan BH, Cameron GM. The isolation of Histoplasma capsulatum from sputum as a diagnostic procedure. The Journal of Laboratory and Clinical Medicine. 1956;**47**(3):499-502

[35] Wheat LJ. Laboratory diagnosis of histoplasmosis: Update 2000. Seminars in Respiratory Infections. Jun 2001;**16**(2):131-140. DOI: 10.1053/srin.2001.24243. PMID: 11521245

[36] Salvin S, Furcolow ML, editors. The Precipitin Test in Human Histoplasmosis. Proc Conference on Histoplasmosis, Pub Health Monograph. Regents of the University of Minnesota, Library; 1956

[37] Pratt PT, Schwartz SO, Ehrlich L. Aspiration biopsy of bone marrow as an aid in diagnosis of histoplasmosis: Report of a case. Archives of Internal Medicine. 1950;**85**(6):893-899

[38] Wheat LJ. Current diagnosis of histoplasmosis. Trends in Microbiology. 2003;**11**(10):488-494

[39] Eissenberg LG, Goldman WE. Histoplasma variation and adaptive strategies for parasitism: New perspectives on histoplasmosis. Clinical Microbiology Reviews. 1991;**4**(4):411-421

[40] Meleney HE. Problems in the histological diagnosis of histoplasmosis. Public Health Monograph. 1956;**70**(39):14-16

[41] Azar MM, Hage CA. Laboratory diagnostics for histoplasmosis. Journal of Clinical Microbiology. 2017;**55**(6):1612-1620

[42] Gaur AH, Giannini MA, Flynn PM, Boudreaux JW, Mestemacher MA, Shenep JL, et al. Optimizing blood culture practices in pediatric immunocompromised patients: Evaluation of media types and blood culture volume. The Pediatric Infectious Disease Journal. 2003;**22**(6):545-552

[43] Murray PR. Comparison of the lysis-centrifugation and agitated biphasic blood culture systems for detection of fungemia. Journal of Clinical Microbiology. 1991;**29**(1):96-98

[44] Santiago AR, Hernández B, Rodríguez M, Romero H. Comparación del método de hemocultivo convencional con el de lisis/centrifugación modificado para el diagnóstico de fungemias. Revista Iberoamericana de Micología. 2004;**21**(4):198-201

[45] Santiago AR, Hernández B, Rodríguez M, Romero H. A comparative study of blood culture conventional method vs. a modified lysis/centrifugation technique for the diagnosis of fungemias. Revista Iberoamericana de Micología. 2004;**21**(4):198-201

[46] Babady NE, Buckwalter SP, Hall L, Le Febre KM, Binnicker MJ, Wengenack NL. Detection of Blastomyces dermatitidis and Histoplasma capsulatum from culture isolates and clinical specimens by use of real-time PCR. Journal of Clinical Microbiology. 2011;**49**(9):3204-3208

[47] Brilhante R, Guedes G, Riello G, Ribeiro J, Alencar L, Bandeira S, et al. RYP1 gene as a target for 556 molecular diagnosis of histoplasmosis. Journal of Microbiological Methods. 2016;**130**:112-114

[48] Edwards LB, Acquaviva FA, Livesay VT, Cross FW, Palmer CE. An atlas of sensitivity to tuberculin, PPD-B, and histoplasmin in the United States. American Review of Respiratory Disease. Apr 1969;**99**(4):Suppl:1-132. PMID: 5767603

[49] Duncan JT. Tropical African histoplasmosis. Transactions of the Royal Society of Tropical Medicine and Hygiene. Sep 1958;**52**(5):468-474. DOI: 10.1016/0035-9203(58)90135-4. PMID: 13592890

[50] Ram R, Swarnalatha G, Prasad N, Dakshinamurty K. Tuberculosis in renal transplant recipients. Transplant Infectious Disease. 2007;**9**(2):97-101

[51] Wheat J. Endemic mycoses in AIDS: A clinical review. Clinical Microbiology Reviews. 1995;**8**(1):146-159

[52] Bradley G, Pine L, Reeves MW, Moss CW. Purification, composition, and serological characterization of histoplasmin—H and M antigens. Infection and Immunity. 1974;**9**(5):870-880

[53] Huppert M, Adler J, Rice E, Sun S. Common antigens among systemic disease fungi analyzed by two-dimensional immunoelectrophoresis. Infection and Immunity. 1979;**23**(2):479-485

[54] Pine L. Histoplasma antigens: Their production, purification and uses. Contributions to Microbiology and Immunology. 1977;**3**:138-168

[55] Sweet GH, Cimprich RS, Cook AC, Sweet DE. Antibodies in histoplasmosis detected by use of yeast and mycelial antigens in immunodiffusion and electroimmunodiffusion. American Review of Respiratory Disease. 1979;**120**(2):441-449

[56] Zancopé-Oliveira R, Bragg S, Hurst S, Peralta J, Reiss E. Evaluation of cation exchange chromatography for the isolation of M glycoprotein from histoplasmin. Journal of Medical and Veterinary Mycology. 1993;**31**(1):29-41

[57] Azuma I, Kanetsuna F, Tanaka Y, Yamamura Y, Carbonell LM. Chemical and immunological properties of galactomannans obtained from Histoplasma duboisii, Histoplasma capsulatum, Paracoccidioides brasiliensis and Blastomyces dermatitidis. Mycopathologia et mycologia applicata. 1974;**54**(1):111-125

[58] Hamilton A, Bartholomew M, Figueroa J, Fenelon L, Hay R. Evidence that the M antigen of Histoplasma capsulatum var. capsulatum is a catalase which exhibits cross-reactivity with other dimorphic fungi. Journal of Medical and Veterinary Mycology. 1990;**28**(6):479-485

[59] Zancopé-Oliveira RM, Reiss E, Lott TJ, Mayer LW, Deepe GS Jr. Molecular cloning, characterization, and expression of the M antigen of Histoplasma capsulatum. Infection and Immunity. 1999;**67**(4):1947-1953

[60] Gross H, Bradley G, Pine L, Gray S, Green JH, Harrell WK. Evaluation of

histoplasmin for the presence of H and M antigens: Some difficulties encountered in the production and evaluation of a product suitable for the immunodiffusion test. Journal of Clinical Microbiology. 1975;**1**(3):330-334

[61] Jacobson ES, Straus SE. Serologic tests for histoplasmosis. Annals of Internal Medicine. 1983;**98**(4):560-561

[62] Markowitz H. Antibodies in histoplasmosis. Journal of Bacteriology. 1967;**93**(1):40-46

[63] Bahr NC, Antinori S, Wheat LJ, Sarosi GA. Histoplasmosis infections worldwide: Thinking outside of the Ohio River valley. Current Tropical Medicine Reports. 2015;**2**:70-80

[64] Wheat L, Musial C, Jenny-Avital E. Diagnosis and management of central nervous system histoplasmosis. Clinical Infectious Diseases. 2005;**40**(6):844-852

[65] Sood A. Altered resting and exercise respiratory physiology in obesity. Clinics in Chest Medicine. 2009;**30**(3):445-454

[66] Almeida MA, Pizzini CV, Damasceno LS, Muniz MM, Almeida-Paes R, Peralta RHS, et al. Validation of western blot for Histoplasma capsulatum antibody detection assay. BMC Infectious Diseases. 2016;**16**(1):1-8

[67] Richer SM, Smedema ML, Durkin MM, Herman KM, Hage CA, Fuller D, et al. Improved diagnosis of acute pulmonary histoplasmosis by combining antigen and antibody detection. Clinical Infectious Diseases. 2016;**62**(7):896-902

[68] Hage CA, Ribes JA, Wengenack NL, Baddour LM, Assi M, McKinsey DS, et al. A multicenter evaluation of tests for diagnosis of histoplasmosis. Clinical Infectious Diseases. 2011;**53**(5):448-454

[69] Connolly PA, Durkin MM, LeMonte AM, Hackett EJ, Wheat LJ. Detection of histoplasma antigen by a quantitative enzyme immunoassay. Clinical and Vaccine Immunology. 2007;**14**(12):1587-1591

[70] Assi M, Lakkis IE, Wheat LJ. Cross-reactivity in the Histoplasma antigen enzyme immunoassay caused by sporotrichosis. Clinical and Vaccine Immunology. 2011;**18**(10):1781-1782

[71] Bahr NC, Sarosi GA, Meya DB, Bohjanen PR, Richer SM, Swartzentruber S, et al. Seroprevalence of histoplasmosis in Kampala, Uganda. Sabouraudia. 2015;**54**(3):295-300

[72] Zhuang D, Hage C, De Jesus M, Hackett E, Durkin M, Davis TE, et al. Cryptococcal glucoxylomannan does not exhibit cross-reactivity in the MVista Histoplasma antigen enzyme immunoassay. Clinical and Vaccine Immunology. 2008;**15**(2):392-393

[73] Johnson PC, Wheat LJ, Cloud GA, Goldman M, Lancaster D, Bamberger DM, et al. Safety and efficacy of liposomal amphotericin B compared with conventional amphotericin B for induction therapy of histoplasmosis in patients with AIDS. Annals of Internal Medicine. 2002;**137**(2):105-109

[74] Kneale M, Bartholomew JS, Davies E, Denning DW. Global access to antifungal therapy and its variable cost. Journal of Antimicrobial Chemotherapy. 2016;**71**(12):3599-3606

[75] Ocansey BK, Kosmidis C, Agyei M, Dorkenoo AM, Ayanlowo OO, Oladele RO, et al. Histoplasmosis in Africa: Current perspectives, knowledge gaps, and research priorities. PLoS Neglected Tropical Diseases. 2022;**16**(2):e0010111

Chapter 4

Pulmonary Histoplasmosis: Clinical and Imagistic Characteristics

Monica Marc, Ana Adriana Trusculescu, Estera Boeriu and Diana Manolescu

Abstract

Histoplasmosis is a condition caused by infection with a fungus, called *Histoplasma capsulatum*. The fungus can be found in the environment in an inactive form (spores), particularly in soil with great amount of bird or bat droppings. Infection occurs when a person inhales the spores and sometimes it can become aggressive especially when the immunity is low or the person has been in contact with a very high amount of fungi. The magnitude of symptoms correlates with the amount of fungi in contact with the patient. About 90% of patients are usually asymptomatic or presenting very few symptoms. However, in immunosuppressed patients, the infection can spread and affect several organs and systems like eyes, liver, spleen, central nervous system, hematological manifestations, joint manifestations. In patients with pre-existing lung disease chronic pulmonary histoplasmosis is not uncommon.

Keywords: histoplasmosis, symptoms, imagistic, extrapulmonary histoplasmosis, pulmonary histoplasmosis

1. Introduction

The fungus incriminated in pulmonary histoplasmosis is *Histoplasma Capsulatum* (*H. Capsulatum*), a dimorphic organism. Having two forms, the mycelial one is observed at ambient temperatures, while at body temperatures, the inhaled microorganism converts to yeast, which is the case of terminal bronchioles and alveoli [1]. Regarding the epidemiology, the most endemic zones of the world are those with temperate climates such as eastern and southern Europe, eastern Asia, Australia, regions of Africa and in the river valleys of the north and central part of the United States [2].

The immunity to *H. Capsulatum* is cell-mediated by IFN-g production from CD4 T lymphocytes and activated macrophages. The macrophages containing the infection lead to granuloma formation. The immune response is given mainly by IL 12, IFN-g, and tumor factor necrosis (TNF)-a [1].

IntechOpen

2. Methodology

The PubMed platform was used as a search tool to collect medical information about histoplasmosis, and "histoplasmosis, clinical, and imaging features" as keywords. We found several articles from which the proper information was selected.

3. Pulmonary histoplasmosis-framework

Most people exposed to *H. Capsulatum* infection will have a mild, even asymptomatic form of the disease, with up to 90% of cases going undiagnosed. However, those under 2 years old and over 50, considered extreme ages, may develop more severe symptoms, with a febrile syndrome, dyspnea, cough, chest pain, and abdominal pain, approximately 2 weeks after exposure. Frequently, the disease is self-limiting, but in case of inhalation of a large inoculum, diffuse histoplasmosis can occur, with severe manifestations, especially dyspnea [3].

The spectrum of imaging changes found in histoplasmosis shows substantial variability, depending on the patient's immunological status, the amount of inoculum at the time of infection, and the organs or systems involved. The radiological lesion pattern can mimic pathologies much more frequently encountered in medical practice, such as community-acquired pneumonia, tuberculosis, and bronchopulmonary neoplasm, but also other pulmonary fungal diseases, which underlines the difficulty of a prompt and certain diagnosis [4].

At the two opposite poles in terms of imaging diagnosis, we identify cases of subclinical histoplasmosis, in which the chest x-ray is present within normal limits, going up to the acute disseminated form with nodular miliary pattern and diffuse pulmonary distribution, such as systemic damage.

4. Clinical and imaging classification

Pulmonary histoplasmosis can take several forms:

4.1 Acute, subacute, and chronic pulmonary histoplasmosis

If symptoms develop, onset occurs 3–14 days after exposure [5]. Acute is defined as less than 1 month of symptoms, while subacute refers to more than 1 month of symptoms but less than three [6]. Fever, headache, malaise, myalgia, abdominal pain, and chills are common symptoms. Joint pain and skin lesions can occur in 5–6% of patients, mostly in women [7]. Enlarged hilar and mediastinal lymph nodes may present in 5–10% of patients. Broncholithiasis can occur if these nodes calcify and may sometimes erode into the airways, leading to possible hemoptysis, obstructive pneumonia, and the expectoration of stones [6]. Cough, hemoptysis, dyspnea, and/or chest pain may be present and are related to the degree of pulmonary airway compression and circulation. Paratracheal involvement may cause coughing or dyspnea due to compression of the trachea or bronchi. Esophageal compression occurs rarely, causing dysphagia.

Acute pulmonary histoplasmosis characterized by imaging (see **Figure 1**) through pulmonary condensations with peribronchovascular distribution and unsystematized lobar, segmental, or multifocal localization in association with mediastinal and hilar adenopathies, reflects the granulomatous reaction and acute alveolar lesions [8].

HISTOPLASMOSIS: CLINIC AND IMAGING

The images are from the database of the „Victor Babeş" Timişoara

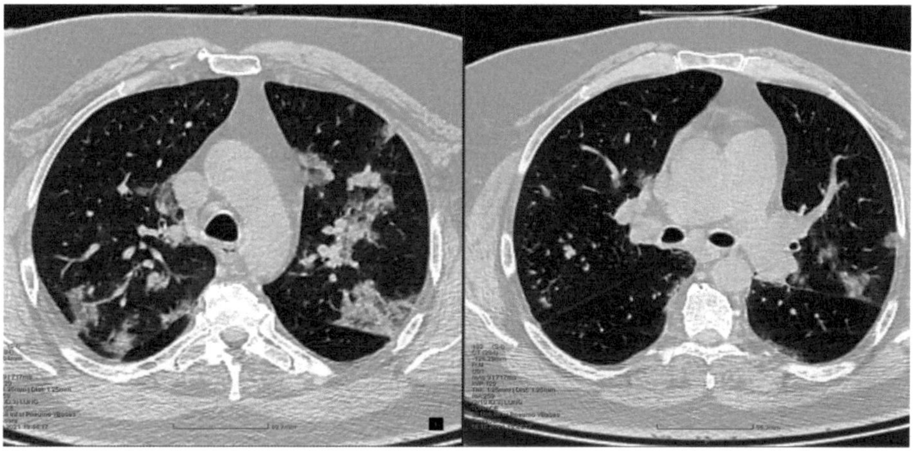

Figure 1.
CT images in the axial plane highlight: (left) the presence of bilateral peribronchovascular infiltrates with associated ground-glass areas; (right) focal centrilobular nodules in the posterior segment of the right upper lobe.

The "tree-in-bud" pattern may be present. Pleural effusion is not characteristic of this disease and does not often appear [4].

Differential diagnoses: Most often, an erroneous diagnosis is established and is often confused with community-acquired or viral pneumonia, which is why antibiotic and antiviral treatment is often administered. Only when the response to this therapy is not expected the clinician raises the suspicion of acute histoplasmosis. It can also be misdiagnosed as other granulomatous pulmonary processes, including mycobacterial, lymphoma, and sarcoidosis.

Within *subacute pulmonary histoplasmosis*, which represents the most frequent form of manifestation of the disease, the chest X-ray can demonstrate a focal area of pulmonary consolidation in association with mediastino-hilar lymphadenopathy (see **Figure 2**). Healing may occur with the formation of a histoplasmoma [9].

Chronic pulmonary histoplasmosis occurs in elderly patients, more often men and smokers. Other risk factors include race (white), pre-existing lung disease, and immunosuppression. It has a slowly progressive nature, and, clinically, it is characterized by symptoms present for over 3 months [3], with an affected general condition, cough, weight loss, dyspnea, and pleuritic chest pain. To these symptoms, increased production of sputum and hemoptysis can be added if the pre-existing lesions are extensive and cavities are present. The objective examination is not specific, non-specific rales are present on auscultation, according to the level of lung damage.

Chronic cavitary histoplasmosis is defined from an imaging point of view by fibro-cavitating lesions located in the upper lobes, most frequently on the background of an emphysematous lung or with underlying structural damage (see **Figure 3**). It can associate the appearance of a "bump," secondary to the mycotic infiltrate superimposed on the level of pre-existing emphysematous bubbles, with a pseudocavitary appearance. The differential diagnosis includes, first of all, pulmonary tuberculosis

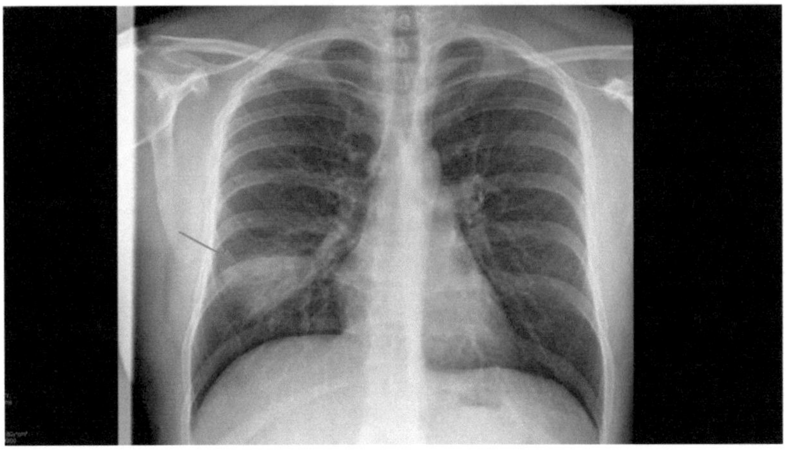

Figure 2.
Chest X-ray (PA) showing a pulmonary opacity in the projection of the right lung base.

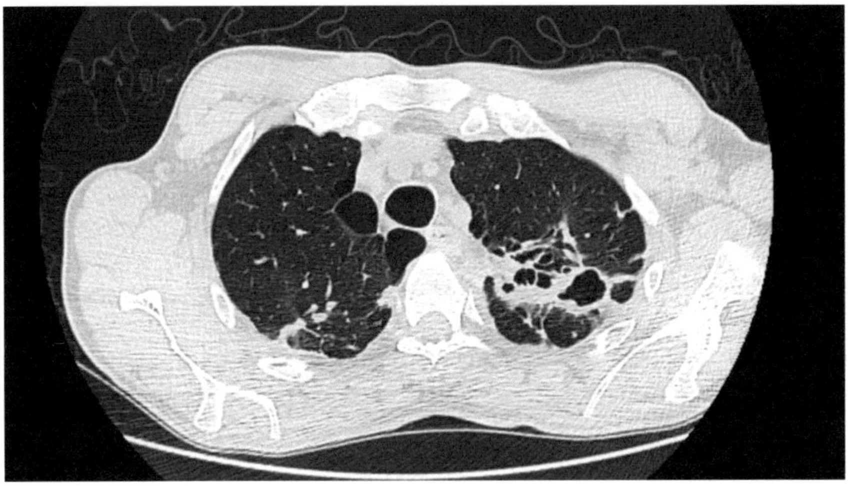

Figure 3.
Axial CT image demonstrates the presence of fibro-cavitation lesions in the apico-posterior segment of the left upper lobe.

with a chronic appearance [8]. This can also be done with other chronic cases of pneumonia, including infections with tuberculous or non-tuberculous mycobacteria, or with other fungal infections: chronic invasive pulmonary aspergillosis, chronic pulmonary coccidioidomycosis or blastomycosis [10].

The *mediastinal and hilar lymph nodes* can often be calcified without necessarily being enlarged. Due to the chronic inflammation, over time, there will be a decrease in lung volume and hilar retraction, with the appearance of fibrosis, loss of parenchyma, and necrosis [10]. The mechanism seems to be immune, through an inadequate response to fungal antigens, rather than through direct fungal aggression [11].

4.2 Chronic progressive disseminated histoplasmosis

It is a severe form, which occurs in immunosuppressed people, for example, patients with HIV, in the AIDS stage with CD4 below 150 cells/μL, and transplant

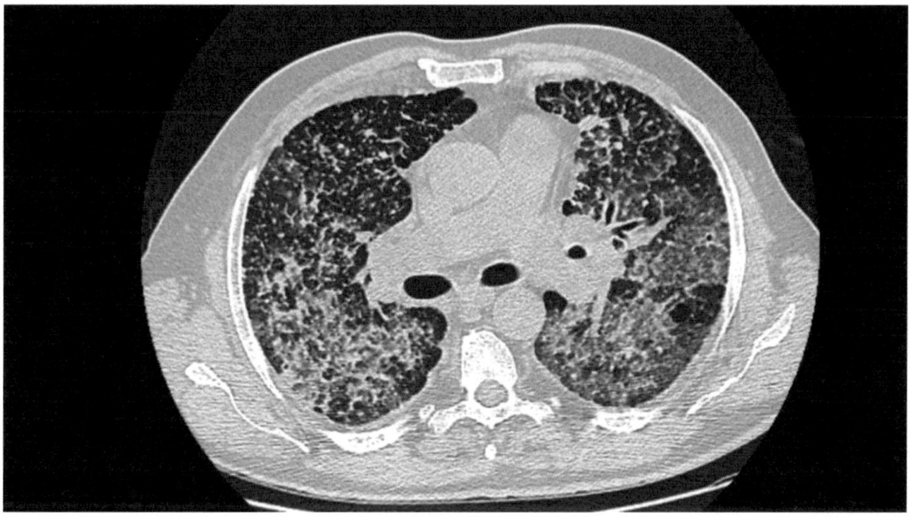

Figure 4.
CT image in the axial plane demonstrates a generalized miliary pattern in both lung fields, with associated ground-glass areas showing a tendency to multifocal condensations.

patients, with malignant hematological pathology. Also, patients who follow various immunosuppressive therapies, such as systemic corticosteroids, tumor necrosis factor antagonists (infliximab, etanercept), or patients exposed to fungi in childhood, are more prone to this severe form. *H. Capsulatum* can remain latent after the initial exposure, and the reactivation can occur years after the initial exposure. The organism can even be transmitted through donated organs [12].

The *disseminated progressive form* presents the following CT characteristics (see **Figure 4**): diffuse pulmonary infiltrates in both lung fields, nodular miliary pattern, or aspect of acute respiratory distress syndrome (ARDS) representing the consequence of uncontrolled fungal proliferation at the level of the reticuloendothelial system with secondary dissemination at the pulmonary, hepato-splenic, gastrointestinal tract and at the hematogenous bone marrow level [9].

4.3 Pulmonary nodules

Pulmonary nodules (see **Figure 5**) from histoplasmosis are frequently detected incidentally, most of them representing the primary healed granulomatous lesion. Histoplasmosis is actually the most common cause of non-cancerous granulomatous nodules and masses in endemic regions [13].

More often, additional investigations are necessary to establish a diagnosis of certainty; the differential diagnosis is made mainly with nodules of malignant etiology; these lesions can mimic bronchopulmonary neoplasm or lung metastases. The differential diagnosis may require the performance of PET CT with 18F-FDG (fluorodeoxyglucose), which will highlight in the subacute phase of the infection lung nodules or masses with a faster reduction of affinity for 18F-FDG compared to associated adenopathies in contrast to proliferative lesions-malignant. Thus, in smoking or ex-smoking patients with nodules over 1 cm, it is necessary to perform a biopsy, either by transthoracic biopsy with a fine needle or by surgical excision. In the case of subcentrimetric nodules, imaging monitoring is recommended. Anti-Histoplasma

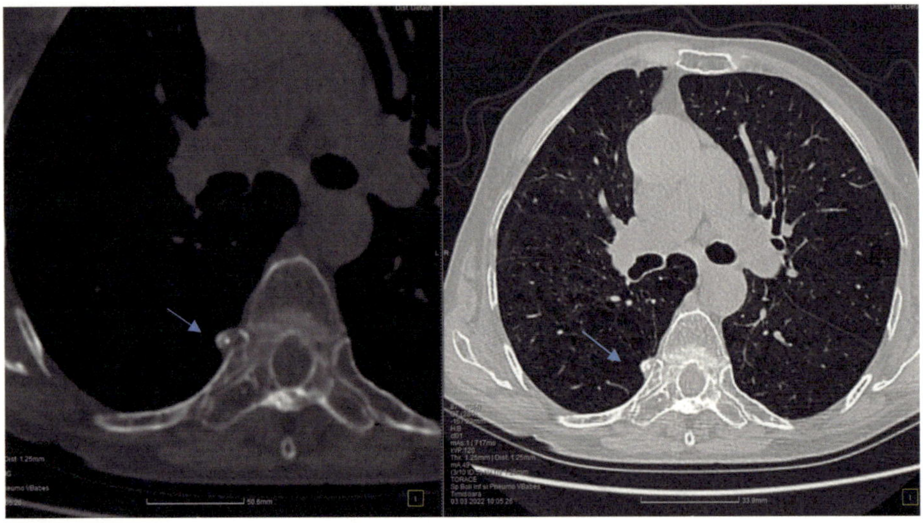

Figure 5.
CT images in the axial plane: (left) solitary pulmonary tissue nodule located in the periphery of the right lower lobe, with central calcification—pathognomonic appearance for histoplasmoma; (right) nodular appearance evident on the lung window.

antibodies can be detected in some patients, but the titers are usually low (1:8–1:16), and antigen tests are mostly negative. In the histopathological examination, both casefied and non-casefied granulomas can be detected. Cultures, even on special media for fungi, are often negative because the organisms are not viable [14, 15].

The *histoplasmoma* represents the solitary healed nodular lesion, with central calcification determining the appearance of a "target" lesion, pathognomonic for histoplasmosis (see **Figure 6**) [16].

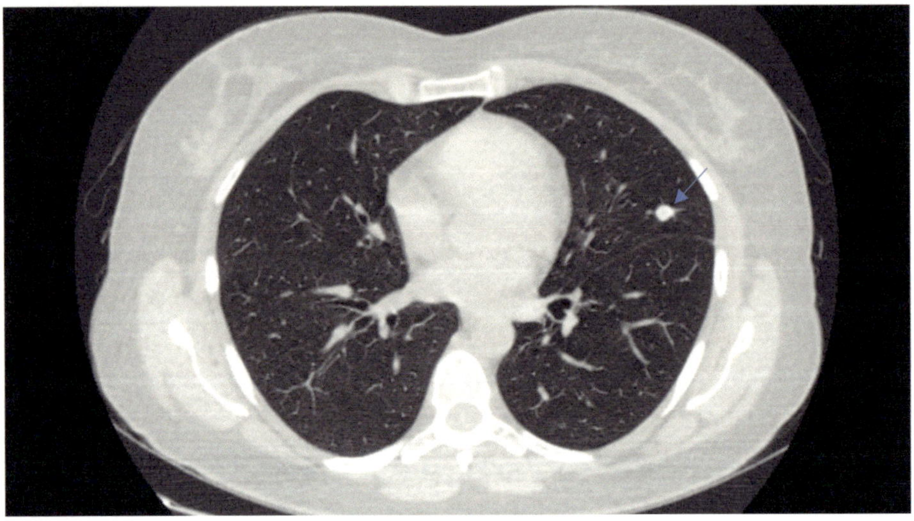

Figure 6.
CT image in the axial plane highlights a lung nodule with soft tissue density, approximately 1 cm in size, with a homogeneous, well-defined, round-oval shape located in the periphery of the left upper lobe.

4.4 Mediastinal histoplasmosis

It can take several forms: mediastinal adenitis, mediastinal granuloma, and fibrosing mediastinitis. The type of damage influences the symptomatology.

4.4.1 Mediastinal adenitis

Most of the time, it is asymptomatic or paucisymptomatic, the most common symptoms being fever and pleuritic chest pain [17, 18]. However, an increase in the ganglia size can cause local obstruction through extrinsic compression, affecting the airways, the superior vena cava, or the esophagus, thus causing different symptoms: dyspnea, swallowing disorders, or cape edema. The radiological image is often suggestive. From an imaging point of view, mediastinal adenitis presents the appearance of mediastinal formation with solid density and homogeneous appearance on CT, in contrast to the heterogeneous appearance of granulomatous mediastinitis.

In isolated cases, pericarditis can also occur. Although this form is often self-limiting, a complete resolution of symptoms occurs after an extended period, from weeks to months. Imaging shows maintenance of the increased dimensions, and their calcification is frequent. Serology is often positive, thus confirming the diagnosis.

In the case of mediastinal adenitis, no specific treatment is recommended, but non-steroidal anti-inflammatory therapy is indicated to reduce pain or fever. However, if the clinical impact is important, specific antifungal treatment with Itraconazole is recommended to prevent disease progression and corticosteroids.

The differential diagnosis is most frequently made with mediastinal granuloma; in mediastinal adenitis, the characteristic is the homogeneous appearance, while in mediastinal granuloma, we have an enlargement of the ganglion with an inhomogeneous appearance [8].

4.4.2 Mediastinal granuloma

It is characterized by forming a semi-liquid adenopathy block, formed by the union of a group of necrotic lymph nodes, most frequently subcarinal and paratracheal. Macroscopically, the necrotic material has the appearance and consistency of a paste, surrounded by a thin capsule (2–3 mm).

As in the case of mediastinal adenitis, mediastinal granuloma can be an accidental discovery, often asymptomatic. Very rarely, in small children, between 2 and 5 years old, it can compress the central airways, the esophagus, or the superior vena cava, as it is known that in these children, the vessels and airways are more flexible [18, 19].

Clinically, it can manifest early after the acute infection, after a few weeks or months, but it can remain subclinical for years when calcifications are detected.

Most of the time, the symptomatology is determined by complications, with adhesion to the neighboring structures and fistulization, with the drainage of the content in the bronchi, pulmonary parenchyma, or esophagus [20]. This liquid usually has a purulent appearance. After the drainage takes place, a new latent phase may appear. The reappearance of symptoms after a certain period can predict an unfavorable evolution over time. Sometimes, drainage to the esophagus can determine the evolution toward sepsis due to the occurrence of retrograde bacterial enteric infection [21, p. 39]. Also, sometimes a fistulization can occur in the pulmonary parenchyma, with the appearance of pneumonic infiltrate or drainage in the pleural or pericardial space, which is extremely rare but urgently requires a surgical pericardial window [22].

Symptomatic mediastinal granuloma requires surgical treatment, but the approach must be made selectively, in the case of adhesions, precisely so as not to cause damage to the surrounding organs. In the case of bacterial superinfections due to fistulization, broad-spectrum antibiotic therapy is necessary in addition to the usual recommended antifungal therapy. Treatment of patients with mediastinal granuloma with itraconazole 200 mg once or twice daily for 6 to 12 weeks in symptomatic patients is reasonable, especially in early mediastinal granuloma, shortly after infection. In the case of asymptomatic mediastinal granuloma, surgical treatment is not recommended [23].

Granulomatous mediastinitis can be the first presentation of histoplasmosis in the form of a mediastinal mass detected on chest X-ray. The CT appearance is of a heterogeneous formation with paratracheal or subcarinal localization, secondary to caseous necrosis at the level of granulomas; internal calcifications may be present [8]. Also, the CT examination can highlight the occurrence of complications: for example, extrinsic compression of the trachea, esophagus, or superior vena cava, respectively fistulization at the mediastinal level, confirmed by the presence of air inclusions at the level of the granuloma. Fistulization at the pulmonary level can be highlighted by a parenchymal infiltrate of the pneumonic type [24].

Fibrosing mediastinitis appears secondary to a chronic inflammatory process with excessive deposits of fibrous tissue at the mediastinal level, which can obstruct the upper respiratory tract and pulmonary vessels. It can be focal (80% of cases, frequently in the case of histoplasmosis) or diffuse (20%). We are thinking of fibrosing mediastinitis in the case of people aged between 20 and 30 years. Although the prevalence is 1 in 100,000 infected patients, it is significant in endemic areas because there are millions of people affected [3]. The symptomatology is determined by the degree of damage to the adjacent structures. The most common symptom is hemoptysis, but the complications can vary depending on the neighboring structures affected [25]. Thus, in unilateral occlusion of the pulmonary artery, pulmonary infarction can be associated with damage to the entire lung. In the case of slow onset of the occlusion, we can have superior vena cava syndrome as a consequence. Most of the time, the damage is unilateral, but patients with fibrosing mediastinitis must be monitored periodically. The CT appearance is variable, with the appearance of a hilar or mediastinal mass (in localized form) or with a fibrosing infiltrative appearance (in diffuse form) with soft tissue density, which obliterates the mediastinal fatty atmosphere and determines the cuffing of the main vessels, with the risk of pulmonary hypertension or obstruction of the superior vena cava [26].

4.5 Forms of extrapulmonary histoplasmosis

In addition to pulmonary manifestations, in some cases (5%) cardiac (pericarditis) [27], skin (erythema multiforme, erythema nodosum) [7], rheumatological (arthritis), ocular manifestations may appear, but these represent a sterile inflammation as part of a systemic response, rather than a disseminated disease.

4.5.1 Progressive disseminated histoplasmosis and meningitis

Approximately 5–20% of patients have CNS involvement. This could include a mass lesion, encephalopathy, and meningitis. Medical therapy is initiated for all patients with progressive disseminated histoplasmosis and meningitis [2].

4.5.2 Cardiac histoplasmosis

Immediate procedural intervention is practiced when there is hemodynamic and respiratory decompensation due to pericardial or pleural damage. In severe cases, thoracocentesis or pericardiocentesis is performed in patients with large pleural effusions, respectively, cardiac tamponade [2].

If the pericardiocentesis is insufficient to alleviate the cardiac tamponade, it may be necessary to place the pericardial window.

Endovascular histoplasmosis can lead to valve infection and aneurysm formation, requiring surgical excision of the infected valves and aneurysm repair. In most cases, endovascular histoplasmosis cannot be cured with medical therapy alone.

4.5.3 Cutaneous and rheumatological histoplasmosis

The lesions are self-limiting. Therapy is indicated only in the case of prolonged episodes or in immunosuppressed patients.

4.5.4 Ocular histoplasmosis

It occurs in 1 to 10% of cases [5]. Extensive maculopathy in suspected ocular histoplasmosis requires steroid treatment. Laser photocoagulation treatment may be necessary for patients with the active formation of neovascular membranes due to choroiditis. Excessive growth can lead to progressive vision loss.

Figure 7 summarizes the histoplasmosis clinical classification and high-resolution computer tomography (HRCT) findings.

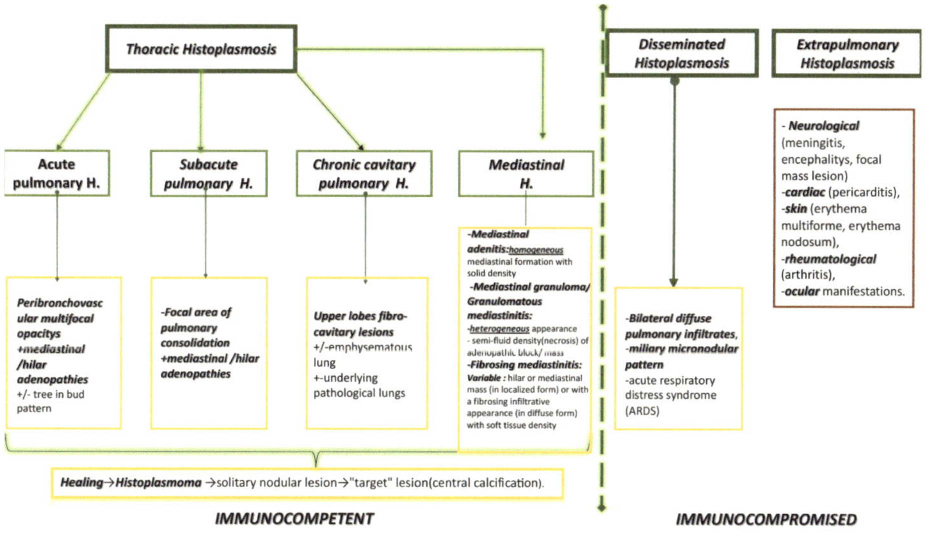

Figure 7.
Histoplasmosis clinical classification and high resolution computer tomography (HRCT) findings.

Author details

Monica Marc[1,2]*, Ana Adriana Trusculescu[1,3], Estera Boeriu[4] and Diana Manolescu[1,5]

1 Center for Research and Innovation in Personalized Medicine of Respiratory Diseases, XIII Department—Pulmonology Discipline, "Victor Babes" University of Medicine and Pharmacy, Timisoara, Romania

2 II Clinic of Pulmonary Diseases, Clinical Hospital of Infectious Diseases and Pneumophtisiology "Dr. Victor Babes", Timisoara, Romania

3 Rehabilitation Clinic of Pulmonary Diseases, Clinical Hospital of Infectious Diseases and Pneumophtisiology "Dr. Victor Babes", Timisoara, Romania

4 Department of Pediatrics, "Victor Babes" University of Medicine and Pharmacy Timisoara, Timișoara, Romania

5 Department of Radiology and Medical Imaging, Clinical Hospital of Infectious Diseases and Pneumophtisiology "Dr. Victor Babes", Timisoara, Romania

*Address all correspondence to: stel_marc@yahoo.com

References

[1] Araúz AB, Papineni P. Histoplasmosis. Infectious Disease Clinics of North America. 2021;**35**(2):471-491. DOI: 10.1016/j.idc.2021.03.011

[2] Jazeela F, Medscape LLC. Histoplasmosis: Background, Pathophysiology, Etiology. New York; 2021. Available from: https://emedicine.medscape.com/article/299054-overview [Accessed: January 4, 2023]

[3] Azar MM, Loyd JL, Relich RF, Wheat LJ, Hage CA. Current concepts in the epidemiology, diagnosis, and management of histoplasmosis syndromes. Seminars in Respiratory and Critical Care Medicine. 2020;**41**(1):13-30. DOI: 10.1055/s-0039-1698429

[4] Sousa C et al. Chest imaging in systemic endemic mycoses. Journal of Fungi Basel Switzerland. 2022;**8**(11):1132. DOI: 10.3390/jof8111132

[5] Hage CA, Wheat LJ, Loyd J, Allen SD, Blue D, Knox KS. Pulmonary histoplasmosis. Seminars in Respiratory and Critical Care Medicine. 2008;**29**(2):151-165. DOI: 10.1055/s-2008-1063854

[6] Tao Le. American Thoracic Society. ATS Review for the Pulmonary Boards American Thoracic Society.pdf—Concise Topic Summaries Ideal for Quick Review Hundreds of Color Images | Course Hero. New York; 2015. Available from: https://www.coursehero.com/file/44441194/ATS-Review-for-the-Pulmonary-Boards-2015-American-Thoracic-Societypdf/ [Accessed: January 4, 2023]

[7] Kauffman CA. Histoplasmosis: A clinical and laboratory update. Clinical Microbiology Reviews. 2007;**20**(1):115-132. DOI: 10.1128/CMR.00027-06

[8] Martin ED, Lassiter RL, Hatley RM, Walters KC. Histoplasmosis presenting as a mediastinal mass. Journal of Pediatric Surgery Case Reports. 2018;**31**:43-45. DOI: 10.1016/j.epsc.2017.11.020

[9] Salzer HJF et al. Diagnosis and management of systemic endemic mycoses causing pulmonary disease. Respiration. 2018;**96**(3):283-301. DOI: 10.1159/000489501

[10] Wheat LJ, Wass J, Norton J, Kohler RB, French ML. Cavitary histoplasmosis occurring during two large urban outbreaks. Analysis of clinical, epidemiologic, roentgenographic, and laboratory features. Medicine (Baltimore). 1984;**63**(4):201-209. DOI:10.1097/00005792-198407000-00002

[11] Goodwin RA et al. Chronic pulmonary histoplasmosis. Medicine (Baltimore). 1976;**55**(6):413-452. DOI: 10.1097/00005792-197611000-00001

[12] Kauffman CA. Histoplasmosis. Clinics in Chest Medicine. 2009;**30**(2):217-225. DOI: 10.1016/j.ccm.2009.02.002

[13] Mukhopadhyay S et al. Pulmonary necrotizing granulomas of unknown cause: Clinical and pathologic analysis of 131 patients with completely resected nodules. Chest. 2013;**144**(3):813-824. DOI: 10.1378/chest.12-2113

[14] Mashburn JD, Dawson DF, Young JM. Pulmonary calcifications and histoplasmosis. The American Review of Respiratory Disease. 1961;**84**(2):208-216. DOI: 10.1164/arrd.1961.84.2.208

[15] Straub M, Schwarz J. The healed primary complex in histoplasmosis. American Journal of Clinical Pathology. 1955;**25**(7):727-741. DOI: 10.1093/ajcp/25.7.727

[16] Torres PPTES, Rabahi MF, Moreira MAC, Santana PRP, Gomes ACP, Marchiori E. Tomographic assessment of thoracic fungal diseases: A pattern and signs approach. Radiologia Brasileira. 2018;**51**(5):313-321. DOI: 10.1590/0100-3984.2017.0223

[17] Goodwin RA, Alcorn GL. Histoplasmosis with symptomatic lymphadenopathy. Chest. 1980;**77**(2): 213-215. DOI: 10.1378/chest.77.2.213

[18] Goodwin RA, Loyd JE, Des Prez RM. Histoplasmosis in normal hosts. Medicine (Baltimore). 1981;**60**(4):231-266. DOI: 10.1097/00005792-198107000-00001

[19] Goodwin RA, Nickell JA, Des Prez RM. Mediastinal fibrosis complicating healed primary histoplasmosis and tuberculosis. Medicine (Baltimore). 1972;**51**(3):227-246. DOI: 10.1097/00005792-197205000-00008

[20] Johnson JA, Loyd JE, Wheat LJ, Netterville JL. A case series and review of histoplasmosis infection in the neck. Archives of Otolaryngology—Head & Neck Surgery. 2010;**136**(9):916-919. DOI: 10.1001/archoto.2010.143

[21] O'Donnell WJ, Kradin RL, Evins AE, Wittram C. Case 39-2004. The New England Journal of Medicine. 2004;**351**(26):2741-2749. DOI: 10.1056/NEJMcpc049030

[22] Gula LJ, Malthaner RA, Quantz MA. Pyopneumopericardium caused by mediastinal granuloma. The Annals of Thoracic Surgery. 2002;**74**(1):241-243. DOI: 10.1016/s0003-4975(02)03609-3

[23] Dines DE, Payne WS, Bernatz PE, Pairolero PC. Mediastinal granuloma and fibrosing mediastinitis. Chest. 1979;**75**(3):320-324. DOI: 10.1378/chest.75.3.320

[24] Garrana SH, Buckley JR, Rosado-de-Christenson ML, Martínez-Jiménez S, Muñoz P, Borsa JJ. Multimodality imaging of focal and diffuse fibrosing mediastinitis. Radiography Review Public Radiological Society of North America. 2019;**39**(3):651-667. DOI: 10.1148/rg.2019180143

[25] Loyd JE, Tillman BF, Atkinson JB, Des Prez RM. Mediastinal fibrosis complicating histoplasmosis. Medicine (Baltimore). 1988;**67**(5):295-310. DOI:10.1097/00005792-198809000-00002

[26] Weerakkody Y. Fibrosing mediastinitis | Radiology Reference Article | Radiopaedia.org. Radiopaedia. Available from: https://radiopaedia.org/articles/fibrosing-mediastinitis [Accessed: January 4, 2023]

[27] Picardi JL, Kauffman CA, Schwarz J, Holmes JC, Phair JP, Fowler NO. Pericarditis caused by histoplasma capsulatum. The American Journal of Cardiology. 1976;**37**(1):82-88. DOI: 10.1016/0002-9149(76)90504-x

Chapter 5

Histoplasmosis: Laboratory Diagnosis

Elena Dumea and Elena Dantes

Abstract

The diagnosis of histoplasmosis is based on clinical, imaging, and laboratory evidence of the disease. The gold standards of laboratory diagnosis are the presence of the fungus in the pathological examination of tissues and its isolation (direct microscopy, histopathology, cytopathology) in mycological culture (4–6 weeks required) by clinical specimens. The antibody test, sometimes negative in immunocompromised patients, must be performed at least four weeks after acute infection to be positive. The antibody test is most useful in subacute and chronic forms of histoplasmosis. The antigen test is the most common method for establishing the diagnosis of acute pulmonary histoplasmosis or progressive disseminated histoplasmosis. The antigen test in urine or serum has good sensitivity, better in bronchoalveolar lavage fluid. There are skin sensitivity tests with low sensitivity that are used only for epidemiologic studies and are not recommended for diagnosis. Molecular diagnosis has improved the sensitivity of clinical specimens. Laboratory PCR assays with different molecular targets have been developed. Currently, the main procedure for molecular diagnosis of histoplasmosis is the application of a rapid DNA probe on a fungus isolated from a culture. This chapter summarizes the currently available tools for the laboratory diagnosis of histoplasmosis, focusing on the complexity of the assays and their performance in different clinical contexts.

Keywords: *Histoplasma*, laboratory diagnostics, microscopy, mycological culture, molecular diagnosis, serological tests, antigen detection tests

1. Introduction

In 2017, the World Health Organization (WHO) created the first list of bacterial priority pathogens (WHO BPPL) and inspired by it, the first list of fungal priority pathogens (WHO FPPL) appeared [1].

The pathogens were classified into three groups according to their ability to cause invasive systemic infections that pose challenges in treatment and/or management or drug resistance: critical, high, and intermediate. *Histoplasma capsulatum* belongs to the high group. Three action areas and strategies were proposed:

1. Improvement of mycological laboratory diagnostic capacity and surveillance, optimization, and standardization of diagnostic tools worldwide;

2. Investment in mycological research, diagnosis, and treatment;

3. Public health interventions with education programs and curricula focused on fungal diseases and priority pathogens.

The geographic distribution of *Histoplasma capsulatum* has changed. It is underestimated because of inadequate public health measures (surveillance and reporting), uneven and unequal access to health care facilities and diagnostic tests (the disease burdens resource-poor regions), climate change, environmental disturbances, improved clinical and laboratory diagnostic detection, and increases in at-risk populations (travelers, immunocompromised patients). Global annual incidence rates for this disease, its distribution, and trends in specific countries or regions are unavailable due to lack of studies. In addition, there is no vaccine, progression to the invasive form is not preventable, access to diagnostics is moderate, and diagnosis for invasive forms is challenging.

Most laboratories have basic tests and only a few have tools such as molecular testing, next-generation sequencing, or other approved tests for histoplasmosis that allow diagnosis of fungal infection when there is high suspicion of the infection.

Diagnosis of Histoplasmosis (HPM) is difficult and requires a multifactorial approach (**Table 1**). Identification of *Histoplasma capsulatum* (*H. capsulatum*) by direct microscopy based on characteristic intracellular yeasts and/or culture isolation of the fungus in biological specimens is the gold standard for diagnosis. However, these tests have their limitations:

a. The low sensitivity, which depends on the clinical form of HPM;

b. The time needed to culture the fungus (4 to 6 weeks), which still requires conversion to the yeast-like form;

c. The need for a level 3 safety laboratory to handle *H. capsulatum*.

In this regard, immunologic methods of antibody and antigen detection in clinical specimens such as serum, plasma, cerebrospinal fluid, urine, and bronchoalveolar lavage (BAL), as well as fungal DNA detection, are options for presumptive diagnosis of HPM. Analytical performance of assays for the diagnosis of histoplasmosis varies depending on disease stage and clinical form (**Table 2**).

2. Antigen detection

The antigen test for histoplasmosis in urine and serum was first developed in 1986 [3], and become an important method for the diagnosis of Histoplasmosis revolutionizing the diagnosis of this disease. The antigen released by the fungal cells can be detected in biological samples: urine, serum, CSF, BAL. Urine antigen detection tests are more sensitive than serum detection tests, results are available within a few hours, they have high sensitivity and specificity, and good negative predictive value.

The first test was a solid-phase radioimmunoassay with the detection of circulating polysaccharide *H. capsulatum* antigen, which was performed after 1989 as an enzyme immunoassay (EIA) [4], with the same sensitivity and specificity but simpler to use.

	Antigen detection	Serologic Test	Molecular methods	Culture	Microscopy (direct and histology)
Specimen	• Urine, serum, CSF, BAL. • Urine antigendetection tests are more sensitive than serum detection tests.	Serum	• Tissues and body fluids, BAL. • Commercially available highly specific molecular tests that allow rapid identification when applied to the culture isolate.	Blood, bone marrow, liver, skin, mucosal lesion, respiratory tract products.	In the microbiology laboratory, *H. capsulatum* can be detected by staining and direct microscopy of body fluids or tissue samples.
Time for positive results after fungal exposure	• Few weeks after exposure. • Is detected in the first few weeks of illness, especially in patients exposed to high levels of fungal inoculum. • Can also be used to evaluate patient response to treatment; it should be below the detection limit if antifungal therapy is successful, and an increase in antigen levels signals relapse.	2 to 6 weeks	• No FDA-approved commercial PCR-based test. • In the future, molecular methods will play an increasingly important role in the diagnosis of HPM.	• 2–3 weeks up to 8 weeks. • The gold standard for diagnosis of HPM is isolation of the fungus in culture and observation of characteristic intracellular yeasts in histopathology.	The presence of *H. capsulatum* yeasts in certain tissues or sterile body fluids (e.g., skin lesions) is indicative of acute infection.
Available within	• Few hours / MVD LFA 1 min/ Alpha *Histoplasma* Antigen EIA- 3 hours • Some tests (MVD EIA) require specimens to be sent to central laboratory.	Depend on laboratory	Hours	• Fungus requires several weeks to grow in standard culture. • The laboratory should have safety level 3 to handle it.	

	Antigen detection	Serologic Test	Molecular methods	Culture	Microscopy (direct and histology)
Tests	• Enzyme-linked immunosorbent assay (ELISA) technique. • The EIA tests MiraVista® • MVD EIA Ag detection. • MVD LFA Alpha *Histoplasma* Antigen EIA, – only test approved by FDA and CE.	• Immunodiffusion (ID)-H and M antigen precipitates. • Complement fixation reaction (CF) -A CF titer ≥1:32 suggest HPM but is not diagnostic, a fourfold increase in antibody titer at least 2 wk. apart. • Enzyme immunoassay (EIA). • Latex agglutination. • Western blot. • IGRAs (Interferon-gamma release assays).	• A real-time PCR assay. • Loop-mediated isothermal amplification (LAMP) (urine).	• Mycelial phase incubation at 25–30°C. • Yeast phase incubation at 37°C. • Conventional blood culture. • Lysis centrifugation system.	• *H. capsulatum* stains poorly with Gram stains, so it is rarely detected by this method. • Fluorescent staining: calcofluor white, that binds chitin in the cell wall of the fungus, is useful for identifying H. *capsulatum* in clinical specimens.
Sensibility and specificity	• Antigen test has high sensitivity and specificity, good negative predictive value. • Depend on clinical form and type test.	• EIA: IgM and IgG antibodies with a sensitivity of 77–96% and a specificity of 92%. • Anti-H antibodies cannot distinguish between the active form and the resolved disease. • EIA more sensitive than ID or CF.	More sensitive and more specific than antigen detection or serologic testing.		
False-positive reactions in urine or serum samples or cross-reactivity	• Cross-reactivity with other mycosis: Blastomycosis, Paraco ccidioidomycosis, Penicilliosis, Talaromycosis, Aspergillosis. • Diagnosis should not be based solely on a positive urine antigen test, further test.	Cross-reactivity with endemic fungi such as Blastomyces dermatitidis.	PCR or LAMP have a lower probability of false-positive.		

Table 1.
Summary of laboratory diagnostic tools.

DOI: http://dx.doi.org/10.5772/intechopen.112411

	Acute pulmonary histoplasmosis	Subacute pulmonary HPM	Chronic pulmonary HPM	Disseminated HPM	HIV and HPM
Antigen tests	*82.8–88.3% [2] • Mira Vista urine antigen sensitivity 83% in acute HPM. • Antigen is detected in approximately 75% of patients with acute pulmonary HPM within the first few weeks of illness, especially in patients exposed to high levels of fungal inoculum.	Only 30.4% in subacute form [2].	• Mira Vista urine antigen sensitivity * 87.5% [2] • In patients with less severe and chronic forms of pulmonary (e.g., cavitary) HPM or in patients with local complications of pulmonary HPM (e.g., mediastinal granuloma), antigen is detected in 10–20% of patients.	• Antigen can be detected in the CSF Mira Vista urine antigen sensitivity is *91.8% in urine • Mira Vista antigen sensitivity in serum is 100%.	• Alpha *Histoplasma* Antigen EIA, (result in 3 hours), has a high sensitivity of 98%, a specificity of 97%, and a negative predictive value of 100% in patients with HIV and HPM and can be performed in individual laboratories. • Alpha *Histoplasma* Antigen detection: in urine at 90% of patients and in serum in 50%. • Antigen detection assays were the most accurate at diagnosing HPM in PLHIV. MVD LFA is a promising tool for point-of-care testing in suspected HPM, especially in people living with HIV/AIDS.
Serology	*64.3–66.7% [2] Anti-M antibodies occur in 80% of patients. Anti-H Ab occurs in less than 20% of cases, appears in severe acute pulmonary HPM. The combination of Ag and Ab improves sensitivity up to 96%.	*95.1% [2]	*83.3% [2] • Anti-M Aboccurs. • Anti-H Ab appeared.	*75% [2] • Serologictest positive at the time of presentation. • Anti-H Ab appeared in disseminated HPM. • Test detection of antibodies to *Histoplasma* in CFS.	• Cross-react with other mycoses: Blastomices, Paracoccidioides, Coccidioides. • −58% sensitivity, greater than 90% specificity. • Antibody detection assays have high specificity, but the sensitivity is poor.

	Acute pulmonary histoplasmosis	Subacute pulmonary HPM	Chronic pulmonary HPM	Disseminated HPM	HIV and HPM
Culture	*0–20% [2] 42% in acute pulmonary HPM.	*53.8% [2]	*66.7% [2]	* 74.2% [2] • In disseminated HPM, specimens collected from the blood, as well as from affected organs such as bone marrow, liver, skin, and mucosal lesions, may result in isolation of *H. capsulatum*. • CSF culture is often negative.	• In PLWHA, up to 90% of respiratory cultures and 50% of blood cultures may be positive. • Antigen and molecular diagnosis assays had greater sensitivity and specificity compared with culture and antibody assays.
Molecular assay			Metagenomic next-generation sequencing (mNGS) on BAL.		Specimen: • respiratory, tissue biopsy, BAL. • blood and bone marrow provided the highest assay sensitivity. • Similar to antigen testing, presented excellent analytical performance for disseminated HPM in PLWHA.
Pathology	*0–42% [2] The presence of *H. capsulatum* yeasts in certain tissues or sterile body fluids (e.g., skin lesions) is indicative of acute infection.	*42.1% [2]	*75% [2] The histopathologic examination is more likely to be positive in the subacute or chronic form than in the acute.	*76.3% [2] The histopathologic examination is more useful in disseminated HPM than in localized pulmonary HPM.	The combination of antigen detection and cytopathology on BAL resulted in a sensitivity of 96.8%, both being rapid diagnostic tools.

***%of diagnostic test for HPM.**

Table 2.
Diagnostic tests depending on clinical form of histoplasmosis.

Two tests based on enzyme-linked immunosorbent assay (ELISA) technique were developed with good diagnostic results but limited availability. Their use is limited to developed endemic areas and is rarely applied in non-endemic regions, probably due to low cost-effectiveness outside these regions.

The EIA tests have been modified several times to provide a quantitative test that can be used in body fluids other than urine and serum, such as CSF or BAL [5], and to avoid exposure of laboratory personnel to radioactivity.

The first test developed was manufactured by MiraVista® (MiraVista Diagnostic, Indianapolis, IN, USA) as a second-generation semi-quantitative test, followed by a third-generation quantitative antigen test. In a multicenter study by Hage et al. [6], the sensitivity and specificity of this test were investigated in different clinical forms of histoplasmosis. They found a sensitivity of 91.8% in urine from patients with disseminated HPM, 87.5% in chronic pulmonary HPM, 83.3% in acute HPM, and only 30.4% in subacute form. In serum samples, the sensitivity of the test was 100% in disseminated HPM. The EIA MiraVista test (MVD EIA) requires specimens to be sent to a central laboratory.

The IMMY® ALPHA ELISA kit (IMMY, Norman, OK) is a two-step immunoenzymatic sandwich test using polyclonal antibodies and can be used for quantitative detection of *Histoplasma* antigens in urine.

Recently, MiraVista Diagnostic developed a lateral flow-based assay for the detection of *Histoplasma* antigens in urine (MVD LFA). It is a single-format, "pregnancy test-like", CE labeled product, that is easy to perform (less than 1 minute to perform the test, 40 minutes to obtain the result), it does not require specialized laboratory equipment or complex infrastructure or highly trained personnel, uses urine with sensitivity and specificity greater than 90% [7, 8], and has a concordance between MVD ELISA and LFA tests of 84%. This technique was first developed for the detection of Aspergillus galactomannan with very good results, and MiraVista released a similar test for the detection of *Histoplasma capsulatum* antigen using an immunochromatographic sandwich dipstick assay. Thus, MVD LFA is a promising tool for point-of-care testing in suspected histoplasmosis, especially in people living with HIV/AIDS (PLWHA). A study conducted to compare MVD LFA and MVD ELISA showed a sensitivity of 96% for both tests and a specificity of 96% for LFA and 77% for ELISA [9].

The only in vitro diagnostic test approved by the FDA and CE is the Alpha *Histoplasma* Antigen EIA, manufactured by Immuno Mycologics (IMMY, Norman, OK, USA). This test, which uses a monoclonal antibody, lasts for 3 hours, has a high sensitivity of 98%, a specificity of 97%, and a negative predictive value of 100% in patients with HIV and histoplasmosis [8], and can be performed in individual laboratories. These rapid antigen tests are very important in low-income areas, with high mortality rates, especially PLWHA.

An ELISA test manufactured by Optimum Imaging Diagnostic for the detection of *Histoplasma* antigenuria was recently studied, with a good sensitivity of 92% but 68% false-positive results [10].

In 2019, WHO included the test for the detection of *Histoplasma* antigens in the second edition of the WHO list of essential in vitro diagnostics [11].

The goal of The International Histoplasmosis Advocacy Group (IHAG) for 2025 is that at least one laboratory in each Latin American country has a rapid test (antigen detection or molecular test) for the diagnosis of histoplasmosis [12].

These tests are very important in patients with HIV and histoplasmosis because their antibody levels are low. In patients with HIV and disseminated histoplasmosis, antigen can be detected in urine in 90% of patients and in serum in 50% [13]. Antigen detection was also useful in bronchoalveolar lavage in PLWHA with *Histoplasma*-related pneumonia [14]. The MVista *Histoplasma* antigen enzyme test was adapted for quantitative detection of antigen in BAL. The combination of antigen detection and cytopathology on BAL resulted in a sensitivity of 96.8, both being rapid diagnostic tools. However, cross-reactivity in patients with Blastomycosis was observed [15].

Antigen is detected in approximately 75% of patients with acute pulmonary histoplasmosis within the first few weeks of illness, especially in patients exposed to high levels of fungal inoculum [16]. In patients with less severe and chronic forms of pulmonary (e.g., cavitary) histoplasmosis or in patients with local complications of pulmonary histoplasmosis (e.g., mediastinal granuloma), antigen is detected in 10–20% of patients [17]. In patients with mediastinal fibrosis or granulomatous mediastinitis, *Histoplasma* antigen cannot be detected in urine or plasma.

In patients with *Histoplasma* meningitis, antigen can be detected in the CSF [18], although CSF culture is often negative. Limited data are available for the use of the antigen test in non-HIV patients with disseminated histoplasmosis, but the test appears to be sensitive for this patient population as well. 92% of patients have antigenuria, but antigen is present in serum in only half of them [17]. There are also no data on the utility of this test in BAL from non-HIV patients.

Antigen detection can also be used to evaluate patient response to treatment; it should be below the detection limit if antifungal therapy is successful, and an increase in antigen levels signals relapse [13]. However, in some patients who have been successfully treated, a low concentration of antigen in the urine may persist for many months [19].

False-positive reactions occur in the majority of urine or serum samples from patients with other mycoses: Blastomycosis (a major diagnostic problem in the United States of America because the endemic areas of Blastomycosis and Histoplasmosis are intermingled and antigen tests show reactivity for both fungi), Paracoccidioidomycosis [20], Talaromycosis, Aspergillosis [5], and less frequently in patients with Coccidioidomycosis [21]. *Aspergillus* galactomannan tests react with *Histoplasma* galactomannan and may be positive in patients with HPM, but patients with *Aspergillosis* do not have false-positive antigen [22].

EIA test results should be interpreted in the appropriate clinical context due to cross-reactivity with other fungal antigens. Diagnosis should not be based solely on a positive urine antigen test; further serologic or/and cultural testing should be performed to confirm the diagnosis. A suspicious false-positive reaction is a positive serum antigen test but a negative urine test. This may also occur in transplant recipients who received thymoglobulin (rabbit antithymocyte globulin) due to human anti-rabbit antibodies that developed in response to thymoglobulin in the second week after administration and disappeared by the eighth week. These antibodies resulted in a false-positive *Histoplasma* antigen test in serum by EIA but not in urine [23].

3. Serologic test

Although antibody detection plays a less important role than antigen detection, antibody tests are useful for diagnosing various forms of HPM. After fungal exposure, anti-*H. capsulatum* antibodies take 2 to 6 weeks to develop, so they are more useful in subacute or chronic HPM than in acute pulmonary HPM. Even if suspicion is high and initial antibody tests are negative, they should be repeated after 1 or 2 months, which may be helpful in diagnosing acute infection. Almost always, patients with disseminated HPM have antibodies to *H. capsulatum* at the time of presentation. Immunocompromised patients may have a negative antibody test (they are unable to respond to *H. capsulatum* antigens and produce antibodies) and may cross-react with other mycoses: *Blastomices*, *Paracoccidioides*, *Coccidioides* [5].

The available serological tests for the detection of *H. capsulatum* antibodies are immunodiffusion (ID), complement fixation reaction (CF), enzyme immunoassay (EIA), latex agglutination, and Western blot. The first three tests are the most commonly performed because of their availability, precision, and convenience. These methods are non-invasive but have their limitations: wide variation in results within a patient, long time for positive results (to develop antibodies after exposure), and cross-reactivity with other endemic fungi such as *Blastomyces dermatitidis* [24].

Immunodiffusion uses an antigen preparation obtained from mycelial culture of *H. capsulatum*, and the presence of antibodies is signaled by the appearance of H and M antigen precipitates on an agar gel. It is widely used in clinical practice, is based on a simple and reliable method, is not expensive, and has good specificity, which is 71–100% higher than the complement fixation method [25].

Anti-M antibodies appear earlier in the course of HPM and may be present for years after the infection has resolved. They occur in acute form (in approximately 80% of patients) or in chronic infection. Thus, a single positive M band cannot distinguish between the active form and the resolved disease [2, 19].

The H-band is much rarer, occurring in less than 20% of cases, and rarely found without an M-band. The H-precipitin band is seen in patients with severe acute pulmonary HPM, with disseminated disease, chronic lung disease, or mediastinal lymphadenopathy over several months. When the infection has resolved, this antibody disappears [26].

The complement fixation assay tests for both antibodies: yeast and mycelium (histoplasmin). A fourfold increase in antibody titer (either of them) is considered positive and indicates active HPM. A CF titer ≥1:32 suggests HPM but it is not diagnostic. Diagnosis should not be based on a single value, as CF antibodies are often present years after infection and a single low CF titer sometimes means that the patient has been exposed to *H. capsulatum* at some point. The CF assay is slightly more sensitive than ID for diagnosing HPM, especially for the yeast phase; the sensitivity of both assays (CF and ID) exceeded 90% in some studies [27]. The CF mycelial antibody is the most specific test but has low sensitivity. The sensitivity of this test is lower in hemolytic or lipemic samples [25].

The development of an easy-to-perform EIA test (MiraVista Diagnostics, Indianapolis, IN, USA) detects IgM and IgG antibodies with a sensitivity of 77–96% and a specificity of 92%.

Comparing these tests using samples from the same patients, the EIA appears to be more sensitive than ID or CF. The utility of the EIA test (or CF and/or ID) is more important in the diagnosis of *Histoplasma* meningitis, as detection of antibodies to *Histoplasma* in CFS may be the only indicator of disease [28].

H. capsulatum can be detected by the latex agglutination test; detection of antibodies to *H. capsulatum* is based on latex connection with histoplasmin. This method has low sensitivity and cross-reactivity with tuberculosis but is inexpensive and specific [24].

Another assay is being investigated to improve the diagnosis of active or latent forms of HPM: Interferon-gamma release assays (IGRAs) [29]. Based on the promising preliminary results, further studies are needed to validate this assay.

Currently, IGRAs have several disadvantages and limitations: short time for sample processing, complex laboratory capacity, and personal experience, high cost for this test.

The combination of methods, antigen and antibody detection can improve sensitivity (up to 96%) for the diagnosis of acute HPM. Similar improved sensitivity has been noted with the combination of antigen detection and cytopathology with the presence of yeast cells consistent with *H. capsulatum* in BAL [30].

4. Molecular methods

For more rapid and accurate detection of *H. capsulatum* in tissues and body fluids, a number of polymerase chain reaction (PCR) methods have been developed: conventional, nested, and real-time PCR (targeting different regions of the *H. capsulatum* genome) with higher sensitivity and specificity, but many of these have been developed in-house. Although these molecular methods are more sensitive and more specific than antigen detection or serologic testing, there is no FDA-approved commercial PCR-based test.

Currently, the main molecular method for diagnosing HPM involves the use of a rapid DNA probe to identify *H. capsulatum* isolated from a variety of culture extracts. A real-time PCR assay has been used to identify *H. capsulatum* in tissue biopsies or at BAL. Other semi-nested PCR assays showed promising results in identifying *H. capsulatum* in blood or tissue from patients in whom HPM was detected.

Loop-mediated isothermal amplification (LAMP) is a nucleic acid amplification technique that can be used in laboratories with limited resources but has some limitations.

Nucleic acid amplification tests (NAAT) such as PCR or LAMP have a lower probability of false-positive results due to other fungi compared to conventional tests.

A reference database has been established for the identification of *H. capsulatum* using matrix-assisted laser desorption ionization time-of-flight mass spectrometry (MALDI-TOF-MS), but limited data are available [31].

Metagenomic next-generation sequencing (mNGS) has been used on BAL to diagnose chronic progressive pulmonary lesions; panfungal PCR can also be used to diagnose HPM, but so far they have only been used for research purposes [32].

Although culture is considered the gold standard test for the diagnosis of HPM, molecular methods may be more sensitive. In the future, molecular methods will play an increasingly important role in the diagnosis of HPM to assist clinicians. Their results are currently limited by the heterogeneity of molecular assays, the targets used, the small number of subjects included in the studies, the different types of specimens tested, and the lack of a standard comparative method, as well as the limited presence of molecular methods in international diagnostic guidelines [33].

More robust multicenter studies including studies in large populations are needed for performance evaluation and validation of these assays in different types of patients or samples.

5. Culture and microbiology stains

The gold standard for diagnosis of HPM is isolation of the fungus in culture and observation of characteristic intracellular yeasts in histopathology.

Culture sensitivity is low, the fungus requires several weeks to grow in a standard culture, and the laboratory should have safety level 3 to handle it.

In the microbiology laboratory, *H. capsulatum* can be detected by staining and direct microscopy of body fluids or tissue samples. *H. capsulatum* stains poorly with Gram stains, so it is rarely detected by this method. Fluorescent staining: calcofluor white, that binds chitin in the cell wall of the fungus, is useful for identifying H. *capsulatum* in clinical specimens.

H. capsulatum can be identified in culture after specimens are inoculated on appropriate medium: Sabouraud dextrose agar, and incubated at 25°C, allowing the fungus to grow.

Growth of the mycelial phase occurs at 25 to 30°C, and colonies usually appear in 2–3 weeks but can take up to 8 weeks. The colony is white to tan in color. After identification of a colony on solid medium, a lactophenol cotton blue test can be performed to determine the morphology of the mold. Initially, septate hyphae are seen, followed by smooth-walled (or less commonly spiny) microconidia (size 2–5 μm), and finally tuberculate macroconidia (size 7–15 μm), which are characteristic of *H. capsulatum* and have a distinct projection on their surface; this development depends on the maturity of the mycelia. Identification of the tuberculate macroconidia strongly suggests *H. capsulatum*, but the fungus belonging to the genus *Sepedonium* may also have such a structure. Therefore, a more definitive, specific test is needed to verify that the mold is *H. capsulatum* before a definitive diagnosis of HPM can be made. There are commercially available, highly specific molecular tests that allow rapid identification when applied to the isolate. There are also more complicated and time-consuming methods, such as the exoantigen test, which is less practical and requires a biosafety level 3 laboratory. They are being replaced by molecular tests.

Yeast-like colonies appear when plates are originally incubated at 37°C, and at microscopy will appear small round narrow-budding yeast. In vitro, the colony is cream-colored and becomes gray with age.

Incubation of the mold at 37°C will transform the mycelia phase into a yeast phase. This has been used in the past as a method to confirm *H. capsulatum* due to its dimorphic nature, but the conversion rate is low and laborious, and therefore, it cannot be used as a diagnostic tool.

There are some factors that influence the sensitivity of cultures to detect *H. capsulatum*: clinical manifestation (the highest positivity (74%) occurs in patients with disseminated chronic cavitary pulmonary HPM followed by acute disseminated pulmonary HPM (42%)) [19], host immunity and disease burden, exposure to a large inoculum for the organism. In other forms of HPM such as mild or moderate acute pulmonary HPM, granulomatous mediastinitis, mediastinal fibrosis, and chronic meningitis, cultures are usually negative. In PLWHA, up to 90% of respiratory cultures and 50% of blood cultures may be positive [25].

In disseminated histoplasmosis, specimens collected from the blood, as well as from affected organs such as bone marrow, liver, skin, and mucosal lesions, may result in isolation of *H. capsulatum*. The average growth time for *H. capsulatum* in blood cultures is between 12 and 15 days [34] and is rarely observed in conventional blood culture systems (where blood culture bottles are incubated only for 5 days). The lysis centrifugation system (isolator tubes) was more sensitive than automated systems for growing *H. capsulatum* from blood [35]. Hyphal forms and large, bizarre yeast shapes are seen on smears of blood cultures, rather than typical small, oval yeasts. If sputum or BAL is sent for culture, the laboratory should be informed of the suspected diagnosis to use selective medium (which adds ammonium hydroxide to the agar surface to increase pH, which is helpful, decreases commensal fungal growth, and increases *H. capsulatum* growth).

6. Histopathology and cytology

The presence of yeast cells consistent with *H. capsulatum* in the tissues allows a presumptive diagnosis of HPM. The organism is sufficiently characteristic to allow diagnosis of proven HPM according to the European Organization for Research and Treatment of Cancer (EORTC) and Mycoses Study Group Education and Research Consortium (MSGERC) consensus guidelines [36]. *H. capsulatum* is a non-encapsulated organism. The "capsule" noted in the original initial description report that gave the species its name was an artifact of tissue processing.

H. capsulatum var. *capsulatum* appears as 2–4 μm narrow, based budding yeast with thin, non-refractile cell walls, stained with Gomori methenamine silver (GMS) or periodic acid-Schiff stains (PAS). Yeasts are typically found intracellularly, phagocytosed in macrophages and histiocytes, often in clusters of many organisms, but can also be found in extracellular spaces, free in tissues. In bone marrow samples, Giemsa staining helps visualize the yeast forms. Wright-Giemsa staining is also applied to peripheral blood and smears to identify intracellular clusters of budding yeasts in patients with disseminated disease. Hematoxylin-eosin (H&E) staining detects *H. capsulatum* when the organism load is very high (otherwise too insensitive).

H. capsulatum var. *duboisii*, the causative agent of African histoplasmosis, is larger (6–12 μm) and easily distinguished; it can be seen as short chains in tissues.

Some organisms can mimic the appearance of *H. capsulatum* in tissues. However, the clinical picture and specific histochemical stains that show a different appearance on histopathological examination help to distinguish *H. capsulatum* from other organisms, such as *Cryptococcus* spp., *Balstomyces* spp., *Candida glabrata*, *Pneumocistis* spp., *Coccidioides* spp., *Talaromyces* spp., *Leishmania* spp., *Toxoplasma gondi*, and *Trypanosoma cruzi*.

In an appropriate clinical context (e.g., acute pneumonia), the presence of *H. capsulatum* yeasts in certain tissues or sterile body fluids (e.g., skin lesions) is indicative of acute infection.

The histopathologic examination requires invasive procedures such as bronchoscopy or biopsies. It is more useful in disseminated HPM than in localized pulmonary HPM and is more likely to be positive in the subacute or chronic form than in the acute [6].

Sometimes non-viable organisms can be found in mediastinal or pulmonary granuloma tissue years after initial infection. Pathology may show incomplete granulomas and/or fibrosis rather than a well-formed pyogranulomatous reaction. Complementary tests such as negative cultures, antigenemia, and luck in symptoms can help distinguish between healed, old disease, and active infection.

Patients with severe disease with diffuse pulmonary infiltrates are likely to have organisms detected on lung biopsy. In patients with granulomatous mediastinitis, the caseous specimen collected from necrotic nodules may contain some yeast-like *H. capsulatum*. In biopsies from patients with fibrosing mediastinitis, organisms are not usually detected in the fibrotic tissue.

Examination of fluids or tissue aspirates for individual cells can provide narrow-based evidence for HPM. Cytologic specimens stained with GMS or PAS show closely spaced budding yeast cells, mainly in macrophages.

It is uncommon to find *H. capsulatum* on cytologic examination of sputum unless it is a burden infection. Cytopathologic examination of BAL has a sensitivity of 50% for acute pulmonary HPM [37]. When cytopathologic examination BAL is combined with fluid antigen testing, the sensitivity increases to 97% [15].

Fine needle aspiration is a method that can provide a cytodiagnosis of HPM when performed on lymph nodes, adrenal glands, or other tissue.

7. Skin reactivity tests

The histoplasmin skin test reagent has been essential in defining the endemic area for *H. capsulatum* and can be used to evaluate previous exposure or latency but not active infection. It was useful in revealing the high frequency of asymptomatic infections in endemic areas.

The skin test has not been useful for diagnosis because it cross-reacts with other fungi (especially *Blastomyces dermatitidis*), produces interference with complement fixation antibody tests, and is insensitive to disseminated infection.

The skin test reagents are no longer commercially available.

8. Conclusions

In North and Latin America, histoplasmosis is the most common endemic fungal infection, but a number of cases have been reported from many areas of the world. In patients who have lived outside endemic areas, a differential diagnosis with HPM should be considered if there is a history of travel or residence in endemic areas.

As a result of climate change, the epidemiology of endemic invasive fungal infections is changing. The exact incidence of HPM throughout the world is still unknown. There is an urgent need to establish a global traceability system to learn more about the diseases.

Disseminated HPM could be diagnosed at an early stage using time-saving methods without cultures, which would reduce hospitalization costs and increase patient survival.

There is an urgent need for newer, faster, and more sensitive diagnostic tools to be available in clinical laboratories around the world to enable faster diagnosis, which plays an important role in improving patient outcomes in the clinic.

Conflict of interest

The authors declare no conflict of interest.

Author details

Elena Dumea[1,2] and Elena Dantes[1,3]*

1 4th Department - Clinical Medical Disciplines, Faculty of Medicine, 'Ovidius' University of Constanta, Constanta, Romania

2 Clinical Infectious Disease Hospital, Constanta, Romania

3 Clinical Hospital of Pneumophtisiology, Constanta, Romania

*Address all correspondence to: elenadumea@yahoo.com

References

[1] WHO Fungal Priority Pathogens List to Guide Research, Development and Public Health Action. 2017. Available from: https://www.who.int/publications/i/item/9789240060241 [Accessed: February 21, 2023]

[2] Azar MM, Hage CA. Clinical perspectives in the diagnosis and management of histoplasmosis. Clinics in Chest Medicine. 2017;**38**(3):403-415. DOI: 10.1016/j.ccm.2017.04.004

[3] Wheat LJ, Kohler RB, Tewari RP. Diagnosis of disseminated histoplasmosis by detection of *Histoplasma capsulatum* antigen in serum and urine specimens. The New England Journal of Medicine. 1986;**314**:84-88. DOI: 10.1056/NEJM198601093140205

[4] Connolly PA, Durkin MM, LeMonte AM, Hackett EJ, Wheat LJ. Detection of *Histoplasma* antigen by a quantitative enzyme immunoassay. Clinical and Vaccine Immunology. 2007;**14**(12):1587-1591. DOI: 10.1128/CVI.00071-07

[5] Azar MM, Hage CA. Laboratory diagnostics for histoplasmosis. Journal of clinical microbiology. 2017;**55**(6):1612-1620. DOI: 10.1128/JCM.02430-16

[6] Hage CA, Ribes JA, Wengenack NL, Baddour LM, Assi M, McKinsey DS, et al. A multicenter evaluation of tests for diagnosis of histoplasmosis. Clinical Infectious Diseases. 2011;**53**(5):448-454. DOI: 10.1093/cid/cir435

[7] Martínez-Gamboa A, Niembro-Ortega MD, Torres-González P, Santiago-Cruz J, Velázquez-Zavala NG, Rangel-Cordero A, et al. Diagnostic accuracy of antigen detection in urine and molecular assays testing in different clinical samples for the diagnosis of progressive disseminated histoplasmosis in patients living with HIV/AIDS: A prospective multicenter study in Mexico. PLoS Neglected Tropical Diseases. 2021;**15**(3):e0009215. DOI: 10.1371/journal.pntd.0009215

[8] Cáceres DH, Gómez BL, Tobón AM, Chiller TM, Lindsley MD. Evaluation of a *Histoplasma* antigen lateral flow assay for the rapid diagnosis of progressive disseminated histoplasmosis in Colombian patients with AIDS. Mycoses. 2020;**63**:139-144. DOI: 10.1111/myc.13023

[9] Cáceres DH, Gómez BL, Tobón ÁM, Minderman M, Bridges N, Chiller T, et al. Validation and concordance analysis of a new lateral flow assay for detection of *Histoplasma* antigen in urine. Journal of Fungi. 2021;7(10):799. DOI: 10.3390/jof7100799

[10] Cáceres DH, Gómez BL, Tobón ÁM, Chiller TM, Lindsley MD. Evaluation of OIDx *Histoplasma* urinary antigen EIA. Mycopathologia. 2022;**187**(1):129-131. DOI: 10.1007/s11046-021-00602-9

[11] Second WHO Model List of Essential in Vitro Diagnostics. Geneva: World Health Organization; 2019 (WHO/MVP/EMP/2019.05). Available from: https://www.who.int/medical_devices/publications/TRS_1022_SAGE_IVD_Second_WML_of_Essential_In_Vitro_Diagnostics/en/. [Accessed: 2023-02-22]

[12] Caceres DH, Adenis A, de Souza JV, Gomez BL, Cruz KS, Pasqualotto AC, et al. The Manaus declaration: Current situation of histoplasmosis in the Americas, report of the II regional meeting of the international histoplasmosis advocacy group. Current

Fungal Infection Reports. 2019;**13**:244-249. DOI: 10.1007/s12281-019-00365-3

[13] Wheat LJ. Improvements in diagnosis of histoplasmosis. Expert Opinion on Biological Therapy. 2006;**6**(11):1207-1221. DOI: 10.1517/14712598.6.11.1207

[14] Wheat LJ, Connolly-Stringfield P, Williams B, Connolly K, Blair R, Bartlett M, et al. Diagnosis of histoplasmosis in patients with the acquired immunodeficiency syndrome by detection of *Histoplasma capsulatum* polysaccharide antigen in bronchoalveolar lavage fluid. American Review of Respiratory Disease. 1992;**145**(6):1421-1424. DOI: 10.1164/ajrccm/145.6.1421

[15] Hage CA, Davis TE, Fuller D, Egan L, Witt JR III, Wheat LJ, et al. Diagnosis of histoplasmosis by antigen detection in BAL fluid. Chest. 2010;**137**(3):623-628. DOI: 10.1378/chest.09-1702

[16] Swartzentruber S, Rhodes L, Kurkjian K, Zahn M, Brandt ME, Connolly P, et al. Diagnosis of acute pulmonary histoplasmosis. Clinical Infectious Diseases. 2009;**49**(12):1878-1882. DOI: 10.1086/648421

[17] Wheat LJ. Laboratory diagnosis of histoplasmosis: Update 2000. Seminars in Respiratory Infections. 2001;**16**(2):131-140. DOI: 10.1053/srin.2001.24243

[18] Wheat LJ, Musial CE, Jenny-Avital E. Diagnosis and management of central nervous system histoplasmosis. Clinical Infectious Diseases. 2005;**40**(6):844-852. DOI: 10.1086/427880

[19] Hage CA, Azar MM, Bahr N, Loyd J, Wheat LJ. Histoplasmosis: Up-to-date evidence-based approach to diagnosis and management. Seminars in Respiratory and Critical Care Medicine. 2015;**36**(5):729-745. DOI: 10.1055/s-0035-1562899

[20] Wheat J, Wheat H, Connolly P, Kleiman M, Supparatpinyo K, Nelson K, et al. Cross-reactivity in *Histoplasma capsulatum* variety *capsulatum* antigen assays of urine samples from patients with endemic mycoses. Clinical Infectious Diseases. 1997;**24**(6):1169-1171. DOI: 10.1086/513647

[21] Kuberski T, Myers R, Wheat LJ, Durkin M, Connolly P, Kubak BM, et al. Diagnosis of coccidioidomycosis by antigen detection using cross-reaction with a *Histoplasma* antigen. Clinical Infectious Diseases. 2007;**44**(5):e50-e54. DOI: 10.1086/511684

[22] Vergidis P, Walker RC, Kaul DR, Kauffman CA, Freifeld AG, Slagle DC, et al. Falsepositive aspergillus galactomannan assay in solid organ transplant recipients with histoplasmosis. Transplant Infectious Disease. 2012;**14**:213-217. DOI: 10.1111/j.1399-3062.2011.00675.x

[23] Wheat LJ, Connolly P, Durkin M, Book BK, Tector AJ, Fridell J, et al. False-positive *Histoplasma* antigenemia caused by antithymocyte globulin antibodies. Transplant Infectious Disease. 2004;**6**(1):23-27. DOI: 10.1111/j.1399-3062.2004.00045.x

[24] Guimarães AJ, Nosanchuk JD, Zancopé-Oliveira RM. Diagnosis of histoplasmosis. Brazilian Journal of Microbiology. 2006;**37**:1-3. DOI: 10.1590/S1517-83822006000100001

[25] Kauffman CA. Histoplasmosis: A clinical and laboratory update. Clinical Microbiology Reviews. 2007;**20**(1):115-132. DOI: 10.1128/CMR.00027-06

[26] Picardi JL, Kauffman CA, Schwarz J, Phair JP, Andersen J, Warth P. Detection of precipitating antibodies to *Histoplasma capsulatum* by counterimmunoelectrophoresis. American Review of Respiratory Disease. 1976;**114**(1):171-176. DOI: 10.1164/arrd.1976.114.1.171

[27] Bauman DS, Smith CD. Comparison of immunodiffusion and complement fixation tests in the diagnosis of histoplasmosis. Journal of Clinical Microbiology. 1975;**2**(2):77-80. DOI: 10.1128/jcm.2.2.77-80.1975

[28] Bloch KC, Myint T, Raymond-Guillen L, Hage CA, Davis TE, Wright PW, et al. Improvement in diagnosis of *Histoplasma* meningitis by combined testing for *Histoplasma* antigen and immunoglobulin G and immunoglobulin M anti-*Histoplasma* antibody in cerebrospinal fluid. Clinical Infectious Diseases. 2018;**66**(1):89-94. DOI: 10.1093/cid/cix706

[29] Datta K, LaRue R, Permpalung N, Das S, Zhang S, Mehta Steinke S, et al. Development of an interferon-gamma release assay (IGRA) to aid diagnosis of histoplasmosis. Journal of clinical microbiology. 2022;**60**(10):e01128-e01122. DOI: 10.1128/jcm.01128-22

[30] Hage CA, Knox KS, Davis TE, Wheat LJ. Antigen detection in bronchoalveolar lavage fluid for diagnosis of fungal pneumonia. Current Opinion in Pulmonary Medicine. 2011;**17**(3):167-171. DOI: 10.1097/MCP.0b013e3283447b60

[31] Valero C, Buitrago MJ, Gago S, Quiles-Melero I, García-Rodríguez J. A matrix-assisted laser desorption/ionization time of flight mass spectrometry reference database for the identification of *Histoplasma capsulatum*. Medical Mycology. 2018;**56**(3):307-314. DOI: 10.1093/mmy/myx047

[32] Chen J, Li Y, Li Z, Chen G, Liu X, Ding L. Metagenomic next-generation sequencing identified *Histoplasma capsulatum* in the lung and epiglottis of a Chinese patient: A case report. International Journal of Infectious Diseases. 2020;**101**:33-37. DOI: 10.1016/j.ijid.2020.09.038

[33] Valero C, Martín-Gómez MT, Buitrago MJ. Molecular diagnosis of endemic mycoses. Journal of Fungi. 2022;**9**(1):59. DOI: 10.3390/jof9010059

[34] Vetter E, Torgerson C, Feuker A, Hughes J, Harmsen S, Schleck C, et al. Comparison of the BACTEC MYCO/F lytic bottle to the isolator tube, BACTEC plus aerobic F/bottle, and BACTEC anaerobic lytic/10 bottle and comparison of the BACTEC plus aerobic F/bottle to the isolator tube for recovery of bacteria, mycobacteria, and fungi from blood. Journal of Clinical Microbiology. 2001;**39**(12):4380-4386. DOI: 10.1128/JCM.39.12.4380-4386.2001

[35] Smith CD, Goodman NL. Improved culture method for the isolation of *Histoplasma capsulatum* and Blastomyces dermatitidis from contaminated specimens. American Journal of Clinical Pathology. 1975;**63**(2):276-280. DOI: 10.1093/ajcp/63.2.276

[36] Donnelly JP, Chen SC, Kauffman CA, Steinbach WJ, Baddley JW, Verweij PE, et al. Revision and update of the consensus definitions of invasive fungal disease from the European Organization for Research and Treatment of cancer and the mycoses study group education and research consortium. Clinical Infectious Diseases. 2020;**71**(6):1367-1376. DOI: 10.1093/cid/ciz1008

[37] Gupta N, Arora SK, Rajwanshi A, Nijhawan R, Srinivasan R. Histoplasmosis: Cytodiagnosis and review of literature with special emphasis on differential diagnosis on cytomorphology. Cytopathology. 2010;**21**(4):240-244. DOI: 10.1111/j.1365-2303.2009.00693.x

Chapter 6

Histoplasmosis: An Overview Treatment of Histoplasmosis

Milena Adina Man, Doina Adina Todea, Nicoleta Ștefania Motoc and Ruxandra-Mioara Rajnoveanu

Abstract

In 2000, the Infectious Diseases Society of America (IDSA) published a clinical practice guideline on managing patients with histoplasmosis and, in 2020, the first global guideline for diagnosing and managing disseminated histoplasmosis in people living with HIV (PLHIV). The classification of pulmonary histoplasmosis is done after clinical presentation and imaging. The optimal treatment depends on the patient's clinical syndrome: acute mild/moderate, acute moderately/severe, chronic cavitary pulmonary, mediastinal lesions, or broncholithiasis. Asymptomatic patients or patients with mild cases of histoplasmosis with symptoms lasting less than four weeks do not usually require antifungal treatment. When necessary, itraconazole is the treatment of choice in mild to moderate acute forms of the disease, often for six weeks. For severe histoplasmosis, amphotericin B is recommended as initial therapy, followed by itraconazole as consolidation therapy. Long-term treatment for at least 12 months is recommended in patients with chronic cavitary histoplasmosis.

Keywords: pulmonary histoplasmosis, *Histoplasma capsulatum*, opportunistic fungal infection, treatment, immunosuppression

1. Introduction

Pulmonary histoplasmosis is a lung disease caused by infection with the fungus *Histoplasma capsulatum* (HC), first described by Dr. Samuel Darling in 1906 [1, 2].

The causative species is comprised of three taxonomic varieties, but only two distinct varieties are known to be pathogens for humans: H. capsulatum var. capsulatum (HC) and H. capsulatum var. duboisii with different geographic distributions, clinical manifestations, and morphologies [3, 4]. The management of the patients varies according to the severity disease and the status of the host's immunity. H Capsulatum is a thermally dimorphic fungus, present as a mold in its natural reservoir, found in soil, caves, and abandoned constructions contaminated with bird droppings. After inhalation of microconidia or mycelial fragments, it converts to a budding yeast form in tissues during the invasive disease [1, 5]. Given this mode of transmission, respiratory infection is the most common manifestation. Yeast multiplies within airspaces and then spreads to adjacent alveoli and subsequently to hilar and mediastinal lymph nodes. In the setting of immunocompetent status, the activated macrophages kill phagocytosed yeast, and even disseminated forms are usually self-limitated [6]. In immunosuppressed patients, the disease severity increase could be fatal and need different treatment' strategies [6, 7].

Although histoplasmosis is well-known in endemic regions and found worldwide in temperate zones of the world, it remains rare in Western Europe [1, 5]. Air currents carry the spores for miles, exposing individuals unaware of contact with the contaminated site, making histoplasmosis a diagnostic challenge for doctors worldwide [7]. Infection usually occurs by inhalation of environmental spores and can occur in both immunocompetent and immunocompromised hosts. Recently, histoplasmosis has raised increasing attention in immunocompetent travelers (the most common endemic mycosis acquired by European travelers) [8]. In this situation, the epidemiological context (visiting endemic county) and type of exposure (bat-infested caves, cleaning of chicken coops, demolition of old buildings, and excavation) could increase the diagnosis suspicion. Therefore, in the presence of clinical and paraclinical pictures, susceptible of pulmonary mycosis histoplasmosis has to be taken into account even in patients that do not have immune disorders and even in non-endemic regions as treatment in some forms is essential. It is important to emphasize that H. capsulatum infection is not transmissible through person-to-person contact [9]. Severity of illness after exposure varies, depending on the exposure intensity, the virulence of the stains and the host immune status. The spectrum of disease ranges from asymptomatic patients to severe, life-threatening disseminated disease, especially in immunocompromised individuals [7, 8]. The population at risk of developing clinically significant histoplasmosis has grown substantially with patients treated with an ever-expanding variety of immunosuppressive medications and/or with immunosuppressive medical conditions [6, 10]. In the general population, primary H. capsulatum infection is asymptomatic in 99% of cases, and only a small proportion of exposed individuals (<0.1%) may develop disseminated disease. Even when it manifests in immunocompetent individuals, the disease is mild, mostly subclinical, often undiagnosed with varying degrees of pneumonia and influenza-like symptoms [11]. On the contrary, in immunocompromised patients with disabled cellular immunity (particularly conditions with compromised cellular immunity affecting T cells), infection cannot be cleared, and the organism continues to reproduce intracellularly and disseminates via lymphatic and hematogenous circulation, cumulating in a state called disseminated histoplasmosis [2]. Dissemination may involve various organs, including the oropharynx, lung, lymph nodes, liver, spleen, skin, brain, and adrenal glands. Considering these different kinds of histoplamosis manifestation with varied symptoms, severity, the management and duration of treatment require a personalized approach [10, 11]. Disseminated progressive disease is more frequent in persons with cell-mediated immunological defects like hematological malignancies, HIV, transplant recipients, hepatitis C, HTLV-1, renal failure, prolonged use of corticosteroids, or biological therapies [2, 12]. In these patients, the disease can occur due to primary infection, reinfection, or dissemination of latent foci persisting after remote infection. If reactivation occurs, a large population of immunosuppressed persons would be at risk (approximately 20% of the U.S. population has had prior subclinical histoplasmosis). Reactivation of latent infections may complicate recipients of solid organ transplants and patients receiving immunosuppressive therapy for other reasons [6, 12]. Exposure to *H. capsulatum* does not confer immunity to reinfection [12]. Up to 40% of patients presenting with disseminated histoplasmosis do not have any obvious risk factors [2].

Histoplasmosis could be divided into several clinical forms [11]:

a. histoplasmosis in the normal host, subdivided into asymptomatic primary infection and acute pulmonary infection;

b. chronic pulmonary histoplasmosis (acute disease, after progression from pulmonary infiltrates to fibrosis and finally cavitation);

c. histoplasmosis in the immunocompromised individuals, corresponding to acute or subacute disseminated histoplasmosis;

d. immunologically mediated disease (latent form).

These distinct clinical syndromes vary by clinical course and wide range of presentation, degrees of severity, extent of disease, delay of diagnosis, and radiographic findings. Therefore, treatment depends on the severity of the clinical syndrome as well as the host immune status [11, 13].

2. Treatment options

Multiple organizations have published treatment guidelines for histoplasmosis: the National Institutes of Health (NIH), the Infectious Diseases Society of America (IDSA), and the Centers for Disease Control and Prevention (CDC) in collaboration with the HIV Medical Association (HIVMA) and the IDSA; the American Thoracic Society; and the World Health Organization (WHO)/Pan American Health Organization (PAHO). Recommendations from these four sets of guidelines are similar and are updated when new data or publications might change a prior recommendation or when the panel feels clarification or additional guidance is warranted [6, 7, 10].

2.1 Histoplasmosis treatment in immunocompetent host

In immunocompetent individuals, the disease is usually mild, asymptomatic, or experiences a self-limiting condition with nonspecific symptoms (fever, malaise, chills, weight loss, night sweats, respiratory, rheumatologic, or gastrointestinal symptoms) and may require only symptomatic measures [7, 9, 11]. For most individuals, signs typically resolve without intervention, and only 5% of *Histoplasma* infections are estimated to require clinical management [11, 14].

Disseminated disease although more frequent among immunocompromised patients can be seen occasionally even in immunocompetent patients, when they have traveled in endemic county and have been infected with a large quantity of *H capsulatum*, or have been exposed to a highly virulent strain.

Antifungal treatment is indicated for certain forms of histoplasmosis, including acute moderate to severe histoplasmosis, chronic disease, and extrapulmonary histoplasmosis. The Infectious Diseases Society of America (IDSA) guidelines state that antifungals could be considered for patients with symptoms lasting >1 month [7]. In **Table 1**, we summarized histoplasmosis treatment considering the immune status and disease severity in acute and chronic forms of histoplasmosis.

	Immunocompetent	Imunosupresions (HIV/imunossupresive terapy)
Acute mild asymptomatic	Antifungal treatment is generally not required	
Symptoms lasting >1 month Mild to moderate acute histoplasmosis	**initial therapy** Itraconazole, (200 mg x 3 orally for the first three days) **maintenance regimen** (200 mg orally once or twice daily) for 6 to 12 weeks	Itraconazole 200 mg twice daily after a loading dose of 200 mg three times daily for three days is used to treat mild to moderate histoplasmosis.
Moderately severe to severe progressive disseminated H	**initial treatment:** Liposomal amphotericin B dosed 3 mg/kg/day intravenously, or amphotericin B lipid complex dosed 5 mg/kg/day intravenously, or amphotericin B deoxycholate dosed 0.7 to 1 mg/kg/day intravenously) **Maintenance therapy** followed by itraconazole (200 mg orally three times daily for the first three days, then 200 mg orally twice daily) for a minimum of 12 weeks up to an additional three months (at least six months)	**Induction therapy**: Liposomal amphotericin B, 3.0 mg/kg for two weeks. **Maintenance therapy**: Itraconazole 200 mg twice daily for 12 months (treatment less than 12 months is envisageable when the person is clinically stable, receiving antiretroviral treatment, has suppressed viral load, and the immune status has improved) **Alternative azole options include** • posaconazole 300 mg x2 for 1 day, then 300 mg daily; • voriconazole 400 mg x2 for 1 day, then 200 mg bid; or • the least desirable option, fluconazole 800 mg daily For long-term suppressive therapy, itraconazole. IDSA advises a dose of 200 mg daily, whereas the CDC/NIH recommends 200 mg x2. Alternative options in rank order include posaconazole 300 mg extended-release capsule daily; voriconazole 200 mg x2; or fluconazole 400 mg daily
Acute respiratory distress syndrome	Methylprednisolone (0.5 to 1.0 mg/kg/day intravenously) for one to two weeks	• IRIS while receiving effective antiretroviral therapy at the time of diagnosis should continue it and begin treatment for histoplasmosis with amphotericin B or itraconazole • Intravenous fluids and oxygen therapy • Various anti-inflammatory agents
Chronic Histoplasmosis nodules cavity	**Initial therapy** Oral itraconazole 200 mg orally x 3 for the first three days) **The maintenance dose** (200 mg orally once or twice daily) for at least one year until 24 months	**Initial treatment** Oral itraconazole 200 mg orally x 3 for the first three days) The maintenance dose (200 mg orally once or twice daily) for at least one year until 24 months

Table 1.
Treatment in histoplasmosis considering the immune status and disease severity in acute and chronic histoplasmosis [7, 11, 12, 15].

In vitro activities of current antifungal drugs (the polyene, azole, and echinocandin classes) used clinically have been established for dimorphic fungi [11]. Antifungal treatment is generally not required in mild to moderate diseases if they do not have symptoms for more than four weeks. The initial therapy should be itraconazole, given as a loading dose (200 mg orally three times daily for the first three days) followed by a maintenance dose (200 mg orally once or twice daily) for 6 to 12 weeks [10].

For moderate form to severe progressive disseminated histoplasmosis cases, the IDSA guidelines recommend initial amphotericin B treatment (liposomal amphotericin B dosed 3 mg/kg/day intravenously or amphotericin B lipid complex dosed 5 mg/kg/day intravenously or amphotericin B deoxycholate dosed 0.7 to 1 mg/kg/day intravenously) followed by itraconazole (200 mg orally three times daily for the first three days, then 200 mg orally twice daily) for a minimum of 12 weeks up to an additional three months [2, 7, 11].

Antifungal treatment in non-immunosuppressed patients is suggested for at least six months, although the severity and site of the disease need to be considered before determining the duration of therapy [11].

In patients with severe dyspnea, hypoxemia, and/or development of acute respiratory distress syndrome, the addition of methylprednisolone (0.5 to 1.0 mg/kg/d intravenously) for one to two weeks has been used in some patients with clinical benefit [16, 17].

All patients with chronic pulmonary histoplasmosis should be treated due to most patients` progressive loss of pulmonary function. Oral itraconazole is given as a loading dose (200 mg orally three times daily for the first three days) followed by a maintenance dose (200 mg orally once or twice daily) for at least one year until 24 months because of the substantial risk of relapse (after treatment stopped up to 10 to 20% of patients with chronic pulmonary histoplasmosis could relapse within two years of stopping therapy) [7, 18]. Chronic cavitary pulmonary histoplasmosis developed after the acute form is marked by low-grade chronic symptoms, development of persistent cavitation, pulmonary fibrosis and pulmonary insufficiency [19].

In chronic pulmonary histoplasmosis, the cavities should be monitored with chest radiography, and if they persist over a 2- to 4-month period, antimicrobial treatment is recommended, especially if there are also symptoms [19].

Chest radiography should be performed every six months for the first year and then annually for four years to monitor for relapse. Without therapy, pulmonary function progressively declines to respiratory insufficiency, the disease will progress, and the patients will die [7, 11, 17–19].

More recent series have emphasized that pulmonary nodules are a more common manifestation of chronic histoplasma infection that can persist a long time and should be differentiated from symptomatic patients who have multiple diffuse nodules and require acute pulmonary histoplasmosis treatment [7, 11].

2.2 Histoplasmosis treatment in immunocompromised patients

An immunocompromised state (due to HIV or other sources of immunosuppression) increases the risk of systemic infection with histoplasmosis. In addition, the immune system dysregulation in autoimmunity and immunosuppressive medications increases serious infection risk as histoplasmosis [17, 20].

After invading the lungs, the infection progressively spreads to other organs. Immunocompromised patients are 10 to 15 times more likely to develop a disseminated form of the disease [7, 20, 21]. The disseminated disease is often fatal if it is not promptly recognized, particularly in patients with HIV infection (histoplasmosis is an AIDS-defining condition), stem cell or solid organ transplantation receivers, and requires a high index of suspicion for timely diagnosis and treatment. In HIV-infected patients, symptomatic illness has been observed in 55% of cases of primary histoplasmosis, and progressive disseminated histoplasmosis occurred in 97–100% of cases of symptomatic histoplasmosis before the availability of highly active antiretroviral therapy [6].

Severely immunocompromised patients often present acutely with fever, pancytopenia, severe respiratory distress, circulatory shock, coagulopathy, and multiorgan failure involving the liver and kidneys. In these patients, histoplasmosis is a life-threatening condition that may require a multi-disciplinary approach to care [20]. Patients with mild immune deficiencies produced by several factors (older age, advanced age, alcoholism, diabetes *mellitus*, solid tumors, corticotherapy, or lymphomas) are more prone to develop chronic histoplasmosis [19].

Histoplasmosis in the immunocompromised host has some particularities. One of the more severe forms of the disease, disseminated histoplasmosis, is a progressive extrapulmonary infection often seen in immunocompromised patients (e.g., AIDS, those on immunosuppressive medications, etc.) or at extremes of age.

2.2.1 Histoplasmosis treatment in HIV patients

Histoplasmosis is an AIDS-defining illness presenting as an invasive form [20]. The most frequent disease in these patients is progressive disseminated histoplasmosis (PDH), where the fungus spreads to other body parts, resulting in high mortality if not treated early [19, 20].

Patients with HIV may require life-long therapy depending on CD4 counts and the status of anti-retroviral treatment [7, 10]. The immunosuppression state is a factor that predisposes the infection due to the CD4+ T-lymphocyte-mediated immunity being compromised [19].

In the first few years of the AIDS pandemic, histoplasmosis carried a high risk for mortality because of the lack of efficacy of ketoconazole. Amphotericin B was effective initially, but in 60% cases experienced relapsed after stopped of treatment. Two treatment phases are recommended: initial induction and long-term maintenance therapy [6].

The IDSA recommended treatment is: a one-to-two-week induction therapy, with liposomal amphotericin B, 3 mg/kg/day for severe disease or itraconazole, a 3-day loading dose of 3x200mg, and then long-term maintenance itraconazole therapy, 200 mg daily, for a minimum period of 12 months [7].

The CDC/NIH and WHO/PAHO guidelines recommend induction for two weeks rather than the 1-to-2-week period advised by the IDSA [7, 20].

In the 2021 Guideline Development Group for Diagnosing And Managing Disseminated Histoplasmosis Among People Living With HIV, three recommendations address the induction and maintenance therapy for histoplasmosis among PLHIV. "The preferred treatment for severe or moderately severe disease is liposomal amphotericin B, 3.0 mg/kg for two weeks" (GRADE classified this recommendation as conditional with very-low-certainty evidence).

"For mild and moderate histoplasmosis, the preferred treatments are itraconazole 200 mg twice a day after an initial dose of 200 mg three times per day for three consecutively days" (GRADE classified this recommendation as conditional with very-low-certainty evidence). For maintenance therapy, the recommended doses are itraconazole 200 mg twice daily for 12 months (GRADE classified this recommendation as conditional with very-low-certainty evidence). Shorter treatment duration can be considered in clinically stable patients that receive antiretroviral treatment that suppressed the viral load with improvement in immune status. (GRADE classified this recommendation as conditional with very-low-certainty evidence) [20].

Global guidelines for the diagnosis and management of endemic mycoses recommended L-AmB as the drug of choice for induction therapy for patients with advanced HIV and moderate-to-severe histoplasmosis, or patients who are sufficiently ill to require hospitalization. However, when L-AmB is not available, other AmB formulations are acceptable alternatives [20].

Liposomal or deoxycholate amphotericin B was more effective in AIDS patients with histoplasmosis (excluding those with CNS involvement) than amphotericin B lipid complex, with one-year survival of 81% and 56%, respectively [22, 23].

Alternative azole options recommended by the NIH/CDC include posaconazole 300 mg x2 for one day, then 300 mg daily; voriconazole 400 mg x2 for one day, then 200 mg bid; or the least desirable option, fluconazole 800 mg daily [6].

Global guideline for the diagnosis and management of endemic mycoses, in individuals with less severe disease, voriconazole is not routinely recommended, and fluconazole has a lower success rate than itraconazole and highlighted the fluconazole resistance in patients receiving fluconazole therapy [21, 23].

Isavuconazole is a newer antifungal triazole used for the treatment of both invasive aspergillosis and mucormycosis with in vitro demonstrated activity against *H. capsulatum*. It could be the best alternative to posaconazole because of its excellent sensitivity, including isolates resistant to fluconazole or voriconazole [24].

A recent Cochrane analysis concluded that the optimum maintenance regimen for histoplasmosis had not been determined (no published study has compared <12 months to >12 months of maintenance treatment) but 95% were relapse-free after 1 year for patients treated with itraconazole, 200 or 400 mg daily [25]. Because of potential toxicity and the need for intravascular access, weekly or biweekly amphotericin B deoxycholate has rarely been used [20, 25, 26].

A complex presentation of disseminated histoplasmosis infection involves the central nervous system (CNS). CNS manifestations can include meningitis involving the basilar meninges, acute meningitis, encephalitis, small ring-enhancing lesions, abscess, and stroke due to infected emboli [27]. Meningitis poses additional challenges in treatment. Liposomal amphotericin B for 4–6 weeks, followed by itraconazole for at least one year, is recommended [27, 28]. IDSA guidelines recommend prophylaxis with itraconazole for as long as the CD4 count remains low (> 150/mm$^{3)}$ in areas where the incidence of histoplasmosis is of >10 cases per 100 person-years. When efavirenz and itraconazole are administered together, itraconazole levels fall by 40%, so higher doses are required [7], and thus, their administration should be closely monitorized.

HIV-associated immune reconstitution inflammatory syndrome (IRIS) is an essential early complication of antiretroviral therapy initiation, associated with considerable morbidity and mortality, particularly in patients who start antiretroviral treatment with advanced immunosuppression [29, 30].

Numerous infective and noninfective conditions are associated with IRIS in HIV infection, including histoplasmosis. Some authors described a higher incidence of disseminated histoplasmosis among patients that recently started antiretroviral therapy, suggesting that this treatment can lead to unmasking IRIS [29]. Patients who manifest findings of IRIS while receiving effective antiretroviral therapy at the time of diagnosis should continue it and begin treatment for histoplasmosis with amphotericin B or itraconazole [29].

Supportive management may be required, including intravenous fluids and oxygen therapy. Various anti-inflammatory agents have been used to treat paradoxical and unmasking IRIS, including corticosteroids and nonsteroidal anti-inflammatory drugs (NSAIDs). The role of corticosteroids remains unclear but could be appropriate in patients with more severe manifestations [29, 30].

In 2019, the WHO included *Histoplasma* antigen tests as an essential diagnostic in endemic areas or non-endemic areas as a reference test for imported cases of histoplasmosis, and by 2025, every country should have access to rapid testing for histoplasmosis. Additionally, itraconazole and both formulations of amphotericin B should be available in the public sector [23, 26].

In the first year, levels of antigenuria and antigenemia should be monitored for early diagnosis of failure or relapse. After successful immune reconstitution and an increase in CD4 count (to more than 150/μL), secondary prevention can be stopped if the patient has received a minimum six-month course of antiretroviral treatment and at least 12 months of antifungal therapy, antigen, and blood culture-negative [7, 11, 29]. However, literature data recommend continuing prophylaxis until the clinical and laboratory results normalize [29]. Monitoring drug interaction in patients with HIV under antiretroviral treatment and histoplamosis is necessary, as these interactions are sometimes diminish efficacy and safety in patients taking these drugs, and they are at risk of toxicity or ineffectiveness from drug interactions. This observation might be useful for patients with advanced disease where possible resistant viruses with limited antiretroviral options [31].

2.2.2 Histoplasmosis secondary to immunosuppressive treatment

Histoplasmosis secondary to TNF-α inhibitor therapy requires discontinuation of the tumor necrosis factor-α blocker during antifungal treatment [22, 32, 33].

Pharmacological immunosuppression with TNF-α inhibitor might be reinstituted after an excellent clinical response after 12 months of anti-histoplasmosis therapy and a negative antigen test [23]. Oral itraconazole, as an antifungal for *H. capsulatum*, could inhibit the CYP3A4 pathway and could decrease steroid metabolites [32]. A growing number of biologics targeting cytokines are available, including inhibitors of the pro-inflammatory mediators such as tumor necrosis factor-alpha (anti-TNF α), interleukin (IL)-1b (canakinumab), IL-1R (anakinra), IL-6R (tocilizumab), as well as T-cell co-stimulation (abatacept) and B-cells (rituximab) but with an increased risk for development of opportunistic infections [34]. TNF is essential for the formation of granuloma and the prevention of granulomatous infections such as tuberculosis and histoplasmosis [32, 33].

For long-term suppressive therapy, each of the four guidelines recommends itraconazole. A dose of 200 mg daily is advised by IDSA, whereas the CDC/NIH recommends 200 mg x2. Alternative options in rank order include posaconazole 300 mg extended-release capsule daily; voriconazole 200 mg x2; or fluconazole 400 mg daily [7].

2.2.3 Histoplasmosis in solid organ transplant recipients

In the field of solid organ transplantation (SOT), T-cell immune dysfunction can also be significant, and the infection can be difficult to predict but remains a rare infection in post-transplant settings, even in endemic areas [34].

Solid organ transplant (SOT) recipients and other immunocompromised hosts have a propensity for severe infection, inclusive of extrapulmonary and disseminated disease. The infections in SOT recipients are best categorized as mild, moderate, or severe [35].

Clinical disseminated histoplasmosis in solid organ transplant (SOT) recipients is nonspecific and rare, with the highest risk period in the first year after transplant, although cases have been reported up to 20 years after transplantation [36]. One-third occurred in the first year, and almost half in the first two years after the transplant [34].

Given the low incidence of histoplasmosis in healthy donors and the rarity of reported donor transmission events, routine donor screening is not indicated, nor the pre-transplant screening for histoplasmosis in transplant candidates, nor even in endemic areas [36]. Donor-derived histoplasmosis is rare, but this confirmed transmission has been reported [34]. Even without clear evidence of dissemination, SOT recipients with histoplasmosis should generally be treated as disseminated disease [5].

The American Society of Transplantation (AST) guidelines recommend at least 1 to 2 weeks of amphotericin B and step down to oral itraconazole. ITZ monotherapy could be used in mild to moderate disease, and longer courses of AmB therapy are recommended for patients with central nervous system (CNS) disease (i.e., 4 to 6 weeks). Irrespective of initial disease severity, antifungal therapy should be continued for a minimum of 12 months or more in patients necessitating continued high-level immunosuppression after a relapsed disease or in CNS involvement. Fluconazole (FCZ) or newer-generation azoles, including voriconazole (VCZ), isavuconazole (ISZ), and posaconazole (PCZ), has been used as an alternative in patients with ITZ intolerance [35]. Once the diagnosis of histoplasmosis is made, immunosuppressive medication should be reduced, although the optimal timing and strategy in this regard are unknown [36]. In patients taking concomitant itraconazole and tacrolimus, concentrations should be assessed to ensure that concentrations are within the narrow therapeutic window or to avoid increased tacrolimus serum levels with potential side effects because of excessive immunosuppression and toxicity (nephrotoxicity and neurotoxicity). Additional pharmacokinetic (PK) and drug–drug interaction considerations must be assessed in kidney transplant patients. Treatment of histoplasmosis with L-AmB comes with nephrotoxicity concerns and possible allograft loss. In the presence of subsequent acute kidney injury, treatment with liposomal amphotericin B (L-AmB) should be associated with concomitant administration of renin-angiotensin system blockers, catecholamines, or immunosuppressants, L-AmB doses ≥3.5 mg/kg/day, and serum potassium <3.5 mEq/L immediately before L-AmB administration [37].

2.3 Treatment in particular forms of histoplasmosis

2.3.1 Mediastinal granuloma, mediastinal lymphadenitis, and fibrosing mediastinitis

A relatively rare complication of pulmonary histoplasmosis is mediastinal granuloma, characterized by enlarging mediastinal lymph nodes. No treatment is recommended for patients with asymptomatic mediastinal granuloma because the active infection is no longer present [7, 11].

Most often, the granuloma is symptomatic secondary to compression of adjacent structures (the esophagus, pulmonary vessels, and trachea), and in these situations, itraconazole for 6–12 weeks is prescribed frequently. Surgical resection of obstructive masses should be considered in the setting of obstruction or in whom a fistula to adjacent structures with drainage of necrotic material has occurred [38, 39].

Fibrosing mediastinitis is a rare disorder characterized by an excessive fibrotic reaction in the mediastinum, which results from an exaggerated host response to a prior infection located at mediastinal lymph nodes [39].

The symptoms are due to the vascular, esophageal, and central airway compression, and fibrosing mediastinitis represents the most severe complication of pulmonary histoplasmosis [38].

2.4 Other manifestations of pulmonary histoplasmosis

a. Broncholithiasis occurs when a calcified node adjacent to a bronchus erodes into the bronchus, causing obstruction, inflammation, and subsequent bronchial scarring; antifungal treatment is not necessary unless the presence of massive hemoptysis or fistula formation when bronchoscopy is required [38].

b. A small proportion of patients with acute pulmonary histoplasmosis develop pericarditis as a complication of the infection that responds to treatment with nonsteroidal anti-inflammatory agents [17, 18].

c. Pleural disease is uncommon during pulmonary histoplasmosis except for the exudative, culture-negative pleural effusions associated with

d. Infection of the central nervous system with histoplasmosis was first recognized in an infant in 1934. Central nervous system histoplasmosis occurs in 5 to 10% of individuals with disseminated diseases, not restricted to immunocompromised individuals, with a high rate of relapse (50%), and increased morbidity and mortality (20–40%) [40, 41].

With the development of effective antifungal therapy, histoplasmosis of SNC has been transformed from a universally fatal illness to a manageable condition if diagnosed early. Aggressive and prolonged antifungal therapy is indicated in all cases of CNS histoplasmosis. However, there is no definitive treatment for CNS histoplasmosis [42].

The Infectious Disease Society of America (IDSA) guideline for the treatment of CNS histoplasmosis recommends an initial course of liposomal amphotericin B because it is known to penetrate CNS structure well (5 mg/kg daily for a total of 175 mg/kg over 4–6 weeks) followed by itraconazole (200 mg 2–3 times daily) for at least one year and until resolution of CSF abnormalities, including negative histoplasma antigen [4, 41, 43].

Because of the risk of relapse, it is recommended to re-evaluate CSF parameters before discontinuation of itraconazole at 12 months and should be followed for at least three years for recurrence.

e. Pregnant patients with histoplasmosis should consider efficacy and safety data carefully. Treatment with amphotericin B for a total of 4–6 weeks, since azoles are teratogenic, particularly in the first trimester, is indicated in moderately severe or severe acute pulmonary disease, chronic pulmonary disease, or disseminated disease and any involving the central nervous system [44, 45].

3. Conclusions

Histoplasmosis is an underdiagnosed infection that affects both immunocompromised and healthy individuals, and early diagnosis requires a high clinical suspicion by clinicians. Management decisions in these patients must balance the severity and localization of the disease, the degree of immunosuppression, the necessity of immunosuppression, the interaction of antifungal drugs, the side effect, the tolerance, and the adherence to treatment. Systematically statements and guidelines assist practitioners and patients in making decisions about appropriate health care for specific clinical circumstances.

Conflict of interest

The authors declare no conflict of interest.

Author details

Milena Adina Man[1†], Doina Adina Todea[1†], Nicoleta Ștefania Motoc[1*]
and Ruxandra-Mioara Rajnoveanu[2]

1 Faculty of Medicine, Department of Medical Sciences-Pulmonology, University of Medicine and Pharmacy, Cluj-Napoca, Romania

2 Faculty of Medicine, Department of Medical Sciences-Palliative Care, University of Medicine and Pharmacy, Cluj-Napoca, Romania

*Address all correspondence to: motoc_nicoleta@yahoo.com

† First and second authors had equal contribution.

References

[1] Zhu C, Wang G, Chen Q, He B, Wang L. Pulmonary histoplasmosis in an immunocompetent patient: A case report and literature review. Experimental and Therapeutic Medicine. 2016;**12**:3256-3260. DOI: 10.3892/etm.2016.3774

[2] Doleschal B, Rödhammer T, Tsybrovskyy O, Aichberger KJ, Lang F. Disseminated histoplasmosis: A challenging differential diagnostic consideration for suspected malignant lesions in the digestive tract. Case Reports in Gastroenterology. 2016;**10**(3):653-660. DOI: 10.1159/000452203

[3] Wijaya M, Adawiyah R, Wahyuningsih R. Histoplasmosis: Diagnostic and therapeutic aspect. Indonesian Journal of Tropical and Infectious Disease. 2021;**9**(2):66-78. DOI: 10.20473/ijtid.v9i2.25448

[4] Drak Alsibai K, Couppié P, Blanchet D, Adenis A, Epelboin L, Blaizot R, et al. Cytological and histopathological Spectrum of histoplasmosis: 15 years of experience in French Guiana. Frontiers in Cellular and Infection Microbiology. 2020;**10**:591974. DOI: 10.3389/fcimb.2020.591974

[5] Jha VK, Mahapatra D. Disseminated histoplasmosis masquerading as significant weight loss eight years post renal transplant. Saudi Journal of Kidney Diseases and Transplantation. 2020;**31**(4):868-873. DOI: 10.4103/1319-2442.292324

[6] McKinsey DS. Treatment and prevention of histoplasmosis in adults living with HIV. Journal of Fungi (Basel). 2021;**7**(6):429. DOI: 10.3390/jof7060429

[7] Wheat LJ, Freifeld AG, Kleiman MB, Baddley JW, McKinsey DS, Loyd JE, et al. Infectious Diseases Society of America. Clinical practice guidelines for managing patients with histoplasmosis: 2007 update by the Infectious Diseases Society of America. Clinical Infectious Diseases. 2007;**45**(7):807-825. DOI: 10.1086/521259

[8] Staffolani S, Riccardi N, Farina C, Lo Cascio G, Gulletta M, Gobbi F, et al. Acute histoplasmosis in travelers: A retrospective study in an Italian referral center for tropical diseases. Pathogens and Global Health. 2020;**114**(1):40-45. DOI: 10.1080/20477724.2020.1716517. 4

[9] Kurowski R, Ostapchuk M. Overview of histoplasmosis. American Family Physician. 2002;**66**(12):2247-2252

[10] Mazi PB, Arnold SR, Baddley JW, Bahr NC, Beekmann SE, McCarty TP, et al. Management of Histoplasmosis by infectious disease physicians. Open forum. Infectious Diseases. 2022;**9**(7):ofac313. DOI: 10.1093/ofid/ofac313

[11] Kauffman CA. Histoplasmosis: A clinical and laboratory update. Clinical Microbiology Reviews. 2007;**20**(1):115-132. DOI: 10.1128/CMR.00027-06

[12] Kuate MPN, Ekeng BE, Kwizera R, Mandengue C, Bongomin F. Histoplasmosis overlapping with HIV and tuberculosis in sub-Saharan Africa: Challenges and research priorities. Therapeutic Advances in Infectious Disease. 2021;**8**:20499361211008675. DOI: 10.1177/20499361211008675

[13] Oliveira PB, Abreu MA, Mattos AL. Importance of multidisciplinary approach in diagnosis of histoplasmosis. Anais Brasileiros de Dermatologia. 2016;**91**(3):362-364. DOI: 10.1590/abd1806-4841.20163821

[14] Benedict K, Beer KD, Jackson BR. Histoplasmosis-related healthcare use, diagnosis, and treatment in a commercially insured population, United States. Clinical Infectious Diseases. 2020;**70**(6):1003-1010. DOI: 10.1093/cid/ciz324

[15] Azar MM, Hage CA. Clinical perspectives in the diagnosis and Management of Histoplasmosis. Clinics in Chest Medicine. 2017;**38**(3):403-415. DOI: 10.1016/j.ccm.2017.04.004

[16] Kauffman KA. Diagnosis and Treatment of Pulmonary Histoplasmosis Literature Review Current Through: 2022 [internet]. Accessed from: uptodate.com

[17] Caceres DH, Knuth M, Derado G, Lindsley MD. Diagnosis of progressive disseminated histoplasmosis in advanced HIV: A meta-analysis of assay analytical performance. Journal of Fungi (Basel). 2019;**5**(3):76. DOI: 10.3390/jof5030076

[18] Thompson GR 3rd, Le T, Chindamporn A, Kauffman CA, Alastruey-Izquierdo A, Ampel NM, et al. Global guideline for the diagnosis and management of the endemic mycoses: An initiative of the European Confederation of Medical Mycology in cooperation with the International Society for Human and Animal Mycology. The Lancet Infectious Diseases. 2021;**21**(12):e364-e374. DOI: 10.1016/S1473-3099(21)00191-2

[19] Baker J, Kosmidis C, Rozaliyani A, Wahyuningsih R, Denning DW. Chronic pulmonary histoplasmosis-a scoping literature review. Open forum. Infectious Diseases. 2020;**7**(5):ofaa119. DOI: 10.1093/ofid/ofaa119

[20] Perez F, Caceres DH, Ford N, Ravasi G, Gomez BL, Pasqualotto AC, et al. For the guideline development group for diagnosing and managing disseminated histoplasmosis among people living with Hiv. Summary of guidelines for managing histoplasmosis among people living with HIV. Journal of Fungi (Basel). 2021;**7**(2):134. DOI: 10.3390/jof7020134

[21] Nacher M, Valdes A, Adenis A, Blaizot R, Abboud P, Demar M, et al. Disseminated histoplasmosis in HIV-infected patients: A description of 34 years of clinical and therapeutic practice. Journal of Fungi (Basel). 2020;**6**(3):164. DOI: 10.3390/jof6030164

[22] Huayllani MT, Restrepo DJ, Boczar D, Sisti A, Rinker BD, Manrique OJ, et al. Histoplasmosis of the upper extremities: Clinical case, treatment algorithm, and systematic review. Hand (N Y). 2021;**16**(3):277-284. DOI: 10.1177/1558944720911212

[23] Myint T, Leedy N, Villacorta Cari E, Wheat LJ. HIV-associated histoplasmosis: Current perspectives. HIV AIDS (Auckl). 2020;**12**:113-125. DOI: 10.2147/HIV.S185631

[24] Mazzella A, Stone NRH, Pool ERM, García Mingo A, Bolache S, Wood C. HIV-associated disseminated histoplasmosis successfully treated with isavuconazole consolidation therapy. Medical Mycology Case Reports. 2019;**27**:42-43. DOI: 10.1016/j.mmcr.2019.12.013

[25] he Murray M, Hine P. Treating progressive disseminated histoplasmosis in people living with HIV. Cochrane Database of Systematic Reviews. 2020;**4**(4):CD013594. DOI: 10.1002/14651858.CD013594

[26] Bongomin F, Kwizera R, Denning DW. Getting histoplasmosis on the map of international recommendations for patients with advanced HIV disease. Journal of Fungi (Basel). 2019;**5**(3):80. DOI: 10.3390/jof5030080

[27] Wheat J, Myint T, Guo Y, Kemmer P, Hage C, Terry C, et al. Central nervous system histoplasmosis: Multicenter retrospective study on clinical features, diagnostic approach and outcome of treatment. Medicine (Baltimore). 2018;**97**(13):e0245. DOI: 10.1097/MD.0000000000010245

[28] Hariri OR, Minasian T, Quadri SA, Dyurgerova A, Farr S, Miulli DE, et al. Histoplasmosis with deep CNS involvement: Case presentation with discussion and literature review. Journal of Neurological Surgery Reports. 2015;**76**(1):e167-e172. DOI: 10.1055/s-0035-1554932

[29] Kiggundu R, Nabeta HW, Okia R, Rhein J, Lukande R. Unmasking histoplasmosis immune reconstitution inflammatory syndrome in a patient recently started on antiretroviral therapy. Autopsy & Case Reports. 2016;**6**(4):27-33. DOI: 10.4322/acr.2016.048

[30] Walker NF, Scriven J, Meintjes G, Wilkinson RJ. Immune reconstitution inflammatory syndrome in HIV-infected patients. HIV AIDS (Auckl). 2015;7:49-64. DOI: 10.2147/HIV.S42328

[31] Huet E, Hadji C, Hulin A, Botterel F, Bretagne S, Lévy Y. Therapeutic monitoring is necessary for the association itraconazole and efavirenz in a patient with AIDS and disseminated histoplasmosis. AIDS. 2008;**22**(14):1885-1886. DOI: 10.1097/QAD.0b013e3283097d0f

[32] Brown RA, Barbar-Smiley F, Yildirim-Toruner C, Ardura MI, Ardoin SP, Akoghlanian S. Reintroduction of immunosuppressive medications in pediatric rheumatology patients with histoplasmosis: A case series. Pediatric Rheumatology Online Journal. 2021;**19**(1):84. DOI: 10.1186/s12969-021-00581-7

[33] Suman S, Lenert A. Diagnostic dilemma of disseminated histoplasmosis mimicking Hemophagocytosis Lymphohistiocytosis in patient with rheumatoid arthritis on anti-TNF therapy: Case report and review of the literature. Case Reports in Rheumatology. 2019;**2019**:4169052. DOI: 10.1155/2019/4169052

[34] Assi M, Martin S, Wheat LJ, Hage C, Freifeld A, Avery R, et al. Histoplasmosis after solidorgan transplant. Clinical Infectious Diseases. 2013;**57**(11):1542-1549. DOI: 10.1093/cid/cit593 Epub 2013 Sep 17

[35] Saullo JL, Miller RA. Updates on histoplasmosis in solid organ transplantation. Current Fungal Infection Reports. 2022;**16**(4):165-178. DOI: 10.1007/s12281-022-00441-1

[36] Nel JS, Bartelt LA, van Duin D, Lachiewicz AM. Endemic mycoses in solid organ transplant recipients. Infectious Disease Clinics of North America. 2018;**32**(3):667-685. DOI: 10.1016/j.idc.2018.04.007

[37] Dodds-Ashley E. Management of Drug and Food Interactions with Azole Antifungal Agents in Transplant Recipients. 2023 [Internet] accessed from: https://www.medscape.com/viewarticle/726344_4

[38] Martin ED, Lassiter RL, Hatley RM, Kenneth C. Wal9ters histoplasmosis presenting as a mediastinal mass. Journal of Pediatric Surgery Case Reports. 2018;**31**:43-45, ISSN 2213-5766,. DOI: 10.1016/j.epsc.2017.11.020

[39] Khalid M, Khan I, Rahman Z, Alazzeh A, Youssef D. Fibrosing Mediastinitis: Uncommon life-threatening complication of histoplasmosis. Cureus. 2018;**10**(4):e2532. DOI: 10.7759/cureus.2532

[40] Riddell JIV, Wheat LJ. Central nervous system infection with *Histoplasma capsulatum*. Journal of Fungi. 2019;**5**:70. DOI: 10.3390/jof5030070

[41] Saccente M. Central nervous system histoplasmosis. Current Treatment Options in Neurology. 2008;**10**(3):161-167. DOI: 10.1007/s11940-008-0017-x

[42] Klumpp L, Liu-Young G, Modi F, Jordan J, Shah R. Reactivation of histoplasmosis disseminated into the central nervous system presenting as a stroke. Cureus. 2019;**11**(12):e6525. DOI: 10.7759/cureus.6525

[43] Gonzalez HH, Rane M, Cioci A, et al. Disseminated central nervous system histoplasmosis: A case report. Cureus. 2019;**11**(3):e4238. DOI: 10.7759/cureus.4238

[44] Whitt SP, Koch GA, Fender B, Ratnasamy N, Everett ED. Histoplasmosis in pregnancy: Case series and report of Transplacental transmission. Archives of Internal Medicine. 2004;**164**(4):454-458. DOI: 10.1001/archinte.164.4.454

[45] Gould AP, Winders HR, Stover KR, Bookstaver PB, Griffin B, Bland CM, et al. Less common bacterial, fungal and viral infections: Review of management in the pregnant patient. Drugs Context. 2021;**10**: 2021-2043. DOI: 10.7573/dic.2021-43

Chapter 7

Is Micro and Nanotechnology Helping Us Fight Histoplasmosis?

Filipa Sousa, Domingos Ferreira, Salette Reis and Paulo Costa

Abstract

Histoplasmosis is an airborne systemic infection, with varied clinical manifestations, from asymptomatic infection to disseminated disease with a deadly outcome. Due to a growing number of immunosuppressed people, this mycosis has become more prevalent and thus, a cause for concern within the medical community. In fact, this fungal infection can be quite serious for children, elderly, people who have had an organ transplant, HIV-positive or people taking immunosuppressants. There has been a limited number of research articles suggesting polymeric, metallic, or lipid micro and nanotechnology-based approaches as a potential way to carry antifungal drugs to treat histoplasmosis. These new drug delivery systems present a variety of means of administration, thereby allowing a more targeted treatment to the lungs, skin, or eyes, according to the infection site. In this review, the aim was to explore these new therapies that have been emerging which hold great potential in comparison to regular antifungal treatments, not only due to their safety but also due to their drug release profile.

Keywords: nanotechnology, histoplasmosis, drug delivery, antifungal, spions, liposomes, polymeric nanoparticles

1. Introduction

Histoplasmosis is the most common respiratory fungal disease and displays the highest endemicity in North and South America [1, 2]. Nonetheless, tourism and migration have stimulated the worldwide growth of histoplasmosis in nonendemic areas, for instance, China, South Africa, India, and Southeast Asia [3, 4]. This disease triggers symptoms and signs, such as fever, weight loss, headache, abdominal pain, chills, fatigue, chest discomfort, diarrhea, and dry cough [5–7].

The infection is caused by inhaling aerosols that contain the infecting particles of the dimorphic fungus, *Histoplasma capsulatum* and it affects most frequently the lung [8]. Nevertheless, it can also affect the skin [9–11], and the central nervous system (CNS) causing meningitis [12] or even evolve into a progressive disseminated infection that may trigger an inflammatory response and bring rheumatological and heart complications (pericarditis), with high morbidity rates [13, 14].

Upon spores' inhalation, the mycelial form goes through a dimorphic transition to yeast to infiltrate the host macrophages in almost any organ, granting its intracellular replication and survival [15–17]. Researchers have proved that the *H. capsulatum* yeasts facility on colonizing and adhering to different organ cryosections (lung, spleen, liver, gut, and trachea) is due to a well-known survival strategy of microorganisms: biofilm formation [18–20].

The at-risk population includes immunocompromised patients or those under immunosuppressive or biological regimens, as well as workers with occupational exposure to spore-laden soil [21].

The disease severity spectrum ranges from asymptomatic or mild lung disease to severe pneumonitis with respiratory compromise, depending on inoculum amount, exposure intensity, and host's immunity [9, 14, 15].

Acute or chronic systemic disease may occur and is associated with immunodepression, particularly acquired immunodeficiency syndrome (AIDS) [3]. In fact, disseminated histoplasmosis among AIDS patients is a rapidly progressing, life-threatening illness that requires prompt treatment with antifungal medication [6]. In Latin America, histoplasmosis is often listed as the number one death cause in patients with advanced AIDS [15].

Infectious diseases caused by intracellular microorganisms, such as histoplasmosis, are described as capable of altering host defense mechanisms and hence allowing these microorganisms to survive inside mononuclear phagocytes, such as macrophages and dendritic cells [22]. These kinds of diseases are regarded as medical challenges due to drug–drug interactions during coinfections and resistance emergencies, which evidently narrows available therapies [23].

Currently, the gold standard treatment for moderate-to-severe disseminated histoplasmosis is liposomal amphotericin B (L-AmB) [1, 6]. The liposomal formulation is preferred to the conventional deoxycholate one, due to decreased nephrotoxicity, lower mortality rates in HIV patients, and overall improved clinical success [3, 24].

On the other hand, for mild and moderate forms of infection, the most appropriate choice is itraconazole. Alternatives to itraconazole include posaconazole, fluconazole, ketoconazole, and voriconazole [1, 13].

Considering the hepatoxicity, limited efficacy due to deficient absorption, low bioavailability, drug degradation, long treatment duration, and frequent drug interactions of the traditional antifungal drugs, it is imperative to develop more efficient strategies for this disease, which would be able to overcome these hurdles [8].

The functionalization of nanocarriers for drug delivery has been ceaselessly disclosing its potential as an alternative and versatile technological platform for the management and treatment of intracellular infections caused by fungi from the *H. capsulatum* species [23, 25]. Indeed, the encapsulation of antifungal agents into nanoparticles to selectively target pathogens has shed light on improving treatment's efficacy and efficiency [8]. Some of these novel drug delivery approaches, such as AmBisome® and Visudyne®, are already commercialized and now serve as benchmark treatments and proof-of-concept of the usefulness of nanotechnology in antifungal drug delivery [26–28].

However, between clear written clinical guidelines and actual clinical practice, there is sometimes a huge gap. In Latin America, for instance, the frequent lack of physician awareness about histoplasmosis and the shortage of accessible diagnostic methods translates into thousands of annual deaths amid advanced-HIV patients, which could have been prevented. It is likewise important to stress that the feasibility of implementing some of these novel treatment options, along with the therapeutic drug monitoring that they require, greatly depends on resource availability, which tends to be scarce in impoverished settings [5, 6].

2. Lipid formulations of Amphotericin B

The burden of invasive fungal infections has grown in the last years, leading to higher morbidity and mortality, especially among immunosuppressed individuals. Amphotericin B deoxycholate (AmBD) (**Figure 1**) is still regarded as one of the most important antifungals of the last 60 years and has been the foundation to treat these infections, showing efficient fungicidal activity against candidiasis, cryptococcosis, aspergillosis, histoplasmosis, blastomycosis, coccidioidomycosis, zygomycosis, sporotrichosis, fusariosis, and phaeohyphomycosis [29, 30].

Nonetheless, given the adverse effects in 50–90% of cases, efforts were made to reformulate the first amphotericin B formulation (Fungizone®) with equivalent efficacy yet reduced toxicity.

The commercially available formulations for this effect are Albelcet® (lipid complex), Amphotec® / Amphocil® (colloidal dispersion), and AmBisome® (liposomal formulation) [27, 29]. On account of their superior safety profiles and higher drug therapeutic index, these lipid-based preparations can nowadays be regarded as worthy substitutes for AmBD. Currently, they are first-line therapy for numerous invasive fungal infections in routine medical practice and clinical investigation, for instance, for disseminated histoplasmosis and AIDS, *Candida* meningitis, or endophthalmitis [27, 31–33].

Even in pregnancy, the lipid formulations of AmB are the cornerstone treatment of any invasive fungal infection and deemed as safe. On the contrary, azoles present complications in view of their teratogenicity, embryotoxicity, and of transplacental infection transmission to the fetus, consequently being contraindicated in this group. Their use during pregnancy should be restricted to superficial infections [14, 34].

Currently, only AmBisome® has been evaluated in the treatment of disseminated histoplasmosis [2, 31]. Besides, some case reports have also stressed its clinical efficacy in the rare primary cutaneous form of the disease in immunocompetent patients [9–11].

AmBisome® received its FDA approval in 1997 and is formed of small spherical unilamellar liposomes with a size inferior to 100 nm, where AmB is encapsulated. L-Amb is represented in **Figure 2**. Hydrogenated soy phosphatidylcholine, cholesterol, and phosphatidylglycerol are composition elements of these liposomes [30].

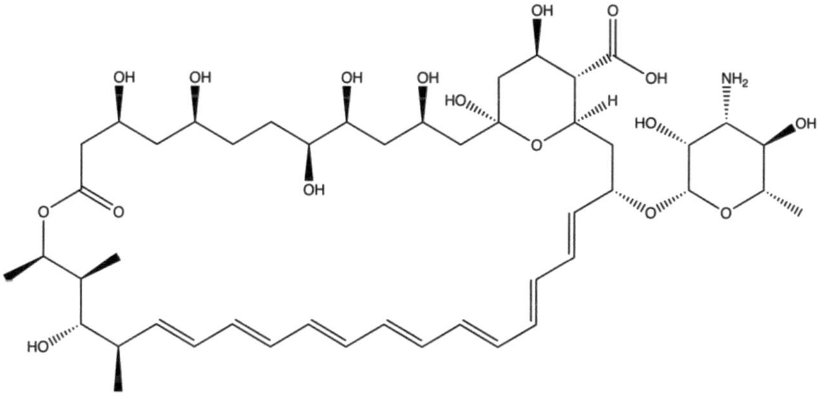

Figure 1.
Chemical structure of amphotericin B ($C_{71}H_{112}NNaO_{21}$). Drawn using ChemDraw Professional 22.0 from PerkinElmer Informatics, Inc.

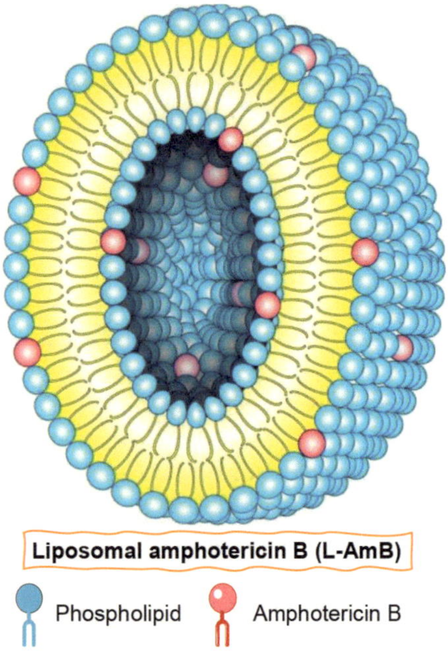

Figure 2.
Schematic representation of liposomal amphotericin B. Parts of the figure were drawn by using pictures from Servier Medical Art. Servier Medical Art by Servier is licensed under a Creative Commons Attribution 3.0 Unported License. (https://creativecommons.org/licenses/by/3.0/).

In a 2002 multicenter randomized, double-blind, prospective clinical trial, with 81 participants, intravenous infusion doses of 3.0 mg/kg of body weight liposomal amphotericin B (L-AmB) and 0.7 mg/kg of AmBD were compared. The purpose was to evaluate both their safety and efficacy for induction therapy of moderate to severe disseminated Histoplasmosis in patients with AIDS [24]. A higher treatment response of 88% was achieved for L-AmB counter to 64% for AmBD, as well as lower mortality rates (2% vs. 13%). Furthermore, nephrotoxicity (assessed through an increase in serum creatinine level) was reported for 9% of patients treated with L-AmB, in opposition to 37% for AmBD, along with fewer infusion-related side effects (25% vs. 63%). Taking all these trial findings into account, L-AmB has clearly revealed to be an upgraded choice to the first standardized treatment AmBD, therefore modifications on therapy recommendations were undertaken after this study. Despite being more costly, L-AmB's attractiveness lies in its less toxic profile, superior efficacy, and improved survival rates for moderate-to-severe invasive histoplasmosis [24, 31].

Nevertheless, clearance rates of fungemia and *H. capsulatum* antigen from serum and urine were alike with the two treatments. For this reason, 2 weeks after the beginning, induction therapy was replaced by itraconazole, for another 10 weeks of consolidation therapy [24, 35].

With the goal of clearly proving the benefits of L-AmB as the initial treatment of moderate-to-severe histoplasmosis, another study was carried out. It comprised two separate closed clinical trials and aimed to compare the clearance of fungal burden (correlated with survival) in patients with disseminated histoplasmosis treated with L-AmB (n = 51) versus itraconazole (n = 59). The clinical response rates were similar: 86% for L-AmB and 85% for itraconazole group. However, after 2 weeks of treatment, fungemia, antigenemia, and antigenuria cleared more rapidly with L-AmB than with itraconazole. This quicker fungemia clearance justifies the use of L-AmB, in opposition to itraconazole, as the initial treatment of moderate-to-severe histoplasmosis [35].

To address the issue of continuously high morbidity and mortality rates brought about by fungal infections, a preclinical study comparing different prophylactic agents was conducted (AmBisome® and Fungizone®). A single high dose of AmBisome® was able to deliver sufficient concentrations of AmB in tissue in immunocompetent and immunosuppressed murine while keeping a safety standard. It effectively inhibited the growth of *Candida albicans* in the kidneys and prevented the growth of *H. capsulatum* in the spleen of mice [36].

3. Drug delivery systems loaded with itraconazole

Itraconazole (**Figure 3**) is an antifungal drug from the azole group, widely used in the treatment of aspergillosis, cryptococcosis, candidiasis, blastomycosis, and mild histoplasmosis. Its action mechanism encompasses the disruption of ergosterol synthesis to avoid the formation of the fungal cell membrane [37, 38].

3.1 Polymeric nanoparticles of itraconazole

Polymeric nanoparticles are capable of not only safely carrying drugs for specific target organs but also of effectively permeating cellular membranes [39].

A striking example of a novel nano-based delivery system is the encapsulation of itraconazole in nanosphere polymeric nanoparticles (NP) based on poly-(lactic-co-glycolic acid) (PLGA) and functionalized with F4/80 antibodies and mannose. The optimized NP was made up of PLGA 75:25 and a mix of surfactants (Kolliphor P188 and vitamin E-TPGS) at pH 5. It showed optimal drug-loading capacity (6.6%), high encapsulation efficiency (80%), and fitted well with the Fickian diffusion model [23]. A schematic representation of this system is outlined in **Figure 4**.

This study has demonstrated increased J774 macrophage uptake *in vitro* and more efficacy in eliminating the *H. capsulatum* on murine macrophages compared with bare NP. Moreover, these NP did not affect the viability in macrophages

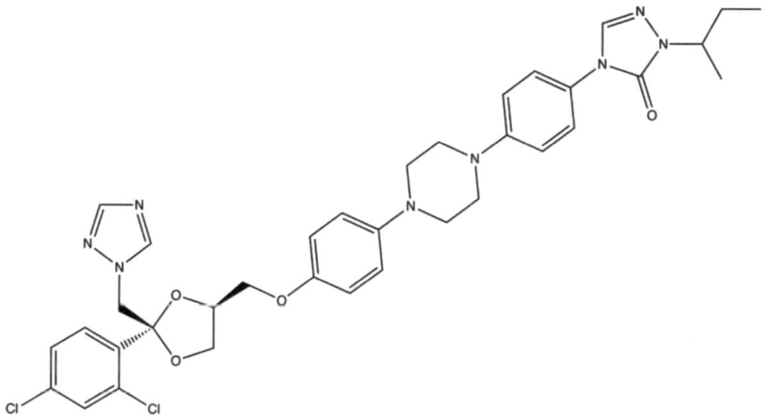

Figure 3.
Chemical structure of itraconazole ($C_{35}H_{38}Cl_2N_8O_4$). Drawn using ChemDraw Professional 22.0 from PerkinElmer Informatics, Inc.

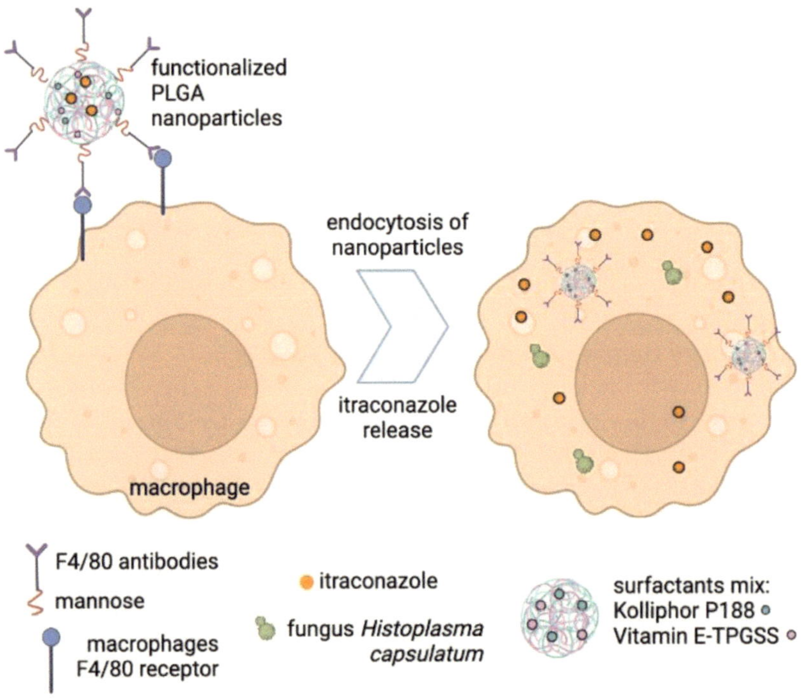

Figure 4.
Schematic representation of the functionalized PLGA NPs loaded with itraconazole and their interaction with F4/80 antibodies receptor in macrophages. Created with BioRender.com.

at different concentrations, which proves they are not cytotoxic. A successful antibody-NP surface binding was achieved while keeping its stability and avoiding aggregation. The 200 nm size is adequate to prevent rapid elimination by the endothelial reticulum system. *H. capsulatum* induces IFN-γ expression in the macrophages and the functionalized NPs developed were able to reduce the expression of this cytokine, emphasizing the role of this antibody as a binding molecule with immunomodulatory properties. In addition, the treatment with these nanoformulations also significantly reduced IL-6 and IL-10 expression compared to free itraconazole. All in all, this research supports the idea that the encapsulation of itraconazole into NP allows a controlled and targeted drug release into macrophages, along with enhanced efficacy and efficiency in battling the fungal intracellular infection [8, 23, 25, 40].

In line with this research was the report of a new polymeric drug delivery system for targeted brain delivery. The authors achieved a stable linkage between RVG29 peptide (a brain-targeting ligand) and itraconazole-loaded albumin nanoparticles by means of the biotin-binding crosslinker streptavidin. This conjugation simplified the intracellular delivery of NPs and enhanced drug distribution in mice brain [41]. Albeit the non-specificity to *H. capsulatum* of either *in vitro* or *in vivo* conducted studies, there is undeniable potential to be exploited herein. In fact, CNS histoplasmosis, despite being rare, is of difficult diagnosis and quickly escalates to disseminated infection with a lower chance of recovery [12].

DOI: http://dx.doi.org/10.5772/intechopen.110544

3.2 Lipid nanoparticles of itraconazole

Nanostructured lipid carriers (NLCs) are attractive drug carriers thanks to their unstructured matrix, which grants enhanced drug loading capacity and long-term drug stability, thereby constituting an upgrade of solid lipid nanoparticles (SLNs) [38, 42].

Itraconazole-NLCs were successfully formulated for brain-targeted delivery. The formulation included Precirol® ATO 5 and Transcutol® HP as lipid phase and Tween 80 and Solutol® HS15 as surfactants. A sustained release was achieved along with an almost double increase in the drug's concentration in the brain, compared to pure itraconazole alone, which in turn showed much lower permeability across the blood–brain barrier [38]. Even though the conducted *in vitro* cellular studies have not targeted *Histoplasma* strains, these itraconazole-NLCs can be further exploited as nanocarriers for brain delivery in SNC histoplasmosis.

4. Drug delivery systems loaded with verteporfin

Verteporfin (**Figure 5**) is a lipophilic benzoporphyrin derivative synthesized from protoporphyrin IX dimethyl ester. It shares several beneficial properties of a photosensitizer: chemical stability, efficient generation of singlet oxygen species, strong absorption of red light at 692 nm, and diminished skin photosensitivity, due to faster body extravasation [43].

4.1 Liposomal formulation of verteporfin

In 2000, both Food and Drug Administration (FDA) and European Medicines Agency (EMA) have approved a liposomal formulation of verteporfin [44]. In fact, encapsulating drugs in liposomes shield drugs from degradation by metabolic enzymes on conjunctiva, cornea, and in tear fluids. Furthermore, liposomes can

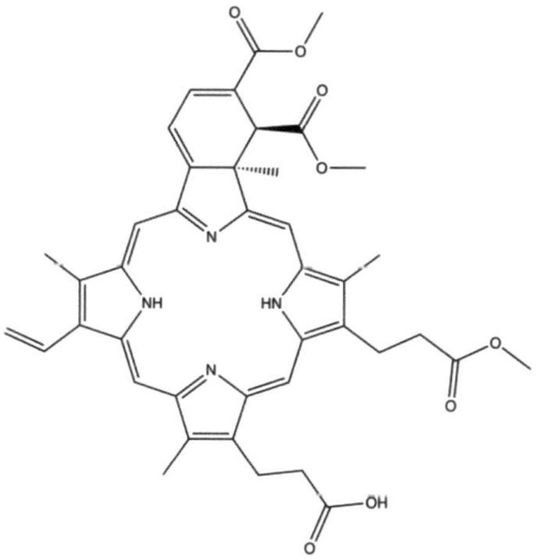

Figure 5.
Chemical structure of verteporfin ($C_{41}H_{42}N_4O_8$). Drawn using ChemDraw Professional 22.0 from PerkinElmer Informatics, Inc.

enhance intraocular penetration and retard the drug's clearance, leading to a higher concentration in the vitreous humor and an increment in the drug's half-life [33].

Since verteporfin is a highly hydrophobic drug, encapsulation in liposomes can control its drug release and enhance its *in vivo* distribution upon intravenous injection [45].

The liposomal formulation was developed by Bausch & Lomb® and is currently marketed by the commercial name Visudyne®. Ophthalmologists consider this formulation a remarkable advance in vision sciences in view of its capability of reducing the magnitude of vision loss for at least 1 year, thus boosting the life quality of these patients [28].

Visudyne® is a light-activated nanomedicine and the first and only clinically approved photosensitizer, being applied in photodynamic therapy (PDT) to eliminate abnormal blood vessels in the eye's retina and choroid (**Figure 6**) [43, 45, 46]. Briefly, it accumulates in these vessels and, when exposed to red light in the presence of oxygen, produces highly reactive free oxygen radicals, which impose local damage to the endothelium and vessel blockage [45, 47, 48]. It has become a milestone in the ophthalmology field for the treatment of patients with subfoveal choroidal neovascularization derived either from age-related macular degeneration, secondary to pathological myopia or from ocular histoplasmosis syndrome [44, 45, 48].

The lipid bilayer of Visudyne® liposomal formulation is made of a synthetic saturated phospholipid DMPC (dimyristoylphosphatidylcholine) and egg yolk phosphatidylglycerol EGPC (comprised of unsaturated multiple species) in the 5:3 ratio [47, 49]. The encapsulation of verteporfin in liposomes was a resourceful way to deliver the drug intravenously, thereby evading the natural predisposition of hydrophobic molecules to self-aggregate in aqueous media [43].

4.2 A theranostic liposome of verteporfin

More recently, in 2020, a group of Brazilian researchers designed a smart theranostic verteporfin-loaded lipid-polymer liposome for PTD. This study proposes the loading of the aforementioned verteporfin liposomes in a theranostic system. Shortly, it consists of lipid-polymer liposomes obtained from DPPC (1,2-dipalmitoyl-sn-glycero-3-phosphatidylcholine) coated with triblock copolymer Pluronic® F127 covalently functionalized with 5 [6]-carboxyfluorescein fluorescent probe. An

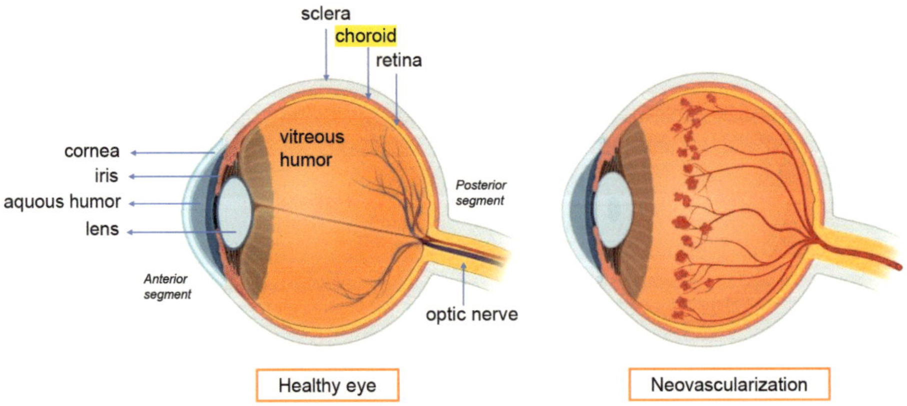

Figure 6.
Comparison between a healthy eye and an eye with choroidal neovascularization, a condition observed in ocular histoplasmosis with the formation of abnormal blood vessels in retina and choroid. Created with BioRender.com.

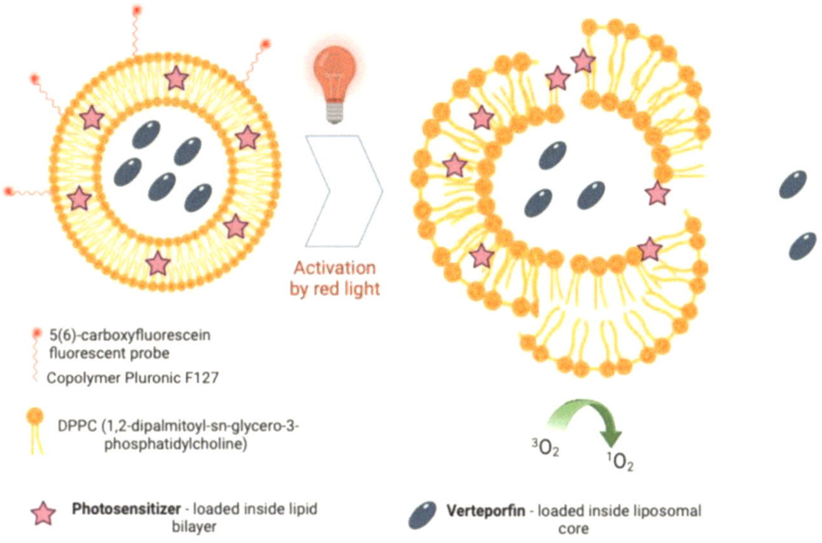

Figure 7.
Schematic representation of a theranostic system to load verteporfin liposomes. Created with BioRender.com.

illustration of this delivery system is depicted in **Figure 7**. This innovative formulation yielded 100 nm vesicles, 0.15 polydispersity index, outstanding stability, and encapsulation efficiency higher than 90%. Despite these encouraging results, the designed system's efficiency was only proven in a glioblastoma cancer cell line, leaving its efficiency in ophthalmic diseases open for further future investigation [49].

5. Magnetic nanoparticles

The insurgence of antimicrobial resistance is the greatest promoter of the fabrication of cutting-edge drug delivery systems. Iron oxide nanoparticles have always merited an outstanding place in drug delivery, thanks to their recognized biomedical importance, precise targeting, and biocompatibility [50].

Bearing this in mind, groups of investigators have recently published promising studies endorsing the development of superparamagnetic, fluorescent, noncytotoxic nano systems with antifungal activity against some fungal strains, namely *H. capsulatum*. In a summarized manner, iron oxide nanoparticles (IONPs) were synthesized using macromolecular stabilizing starch, noteworthy for their biocompatibility and agglomeration prevention. Upon encapsulation with starch, a shift in magnetic behavior takes place, converting the once weakly ferromagnetic IONPs into superparamagnetic (SPIONs) [50, 51]. The SPIONs were successfully incorporated in a fluorescently modified carrier system, enabling not only an easy identification of the system in a living body but also the application of this system in photodynamic therapy. An alarming discovery of this research is that H. *capsulatum* was found to be highly susceptible to the designed nano system in PTD studies, whereas it was resistant to the antifungal griseofulvin [51].

Specific drug targeting to the choroid has lately aroused special interest, on behalf of the rising blindness figures in the aged population and the choroid's unique architecture as one of the most vascularized tissues in the human body.

Magnetic iron oxide nanoparticles stabilized with carboxylic acid, have been covalently functionalized with a recombinant VEGF (vascular endothelial growth factor) permitting the preferential release of the drug into the choroid layer [52]. Albeit the study's core focus was angiogenesis and so they evaluated a monoclonal antibody (bevacizumab), the information conveyed is transposable to histoplasmosis infection. As a matter of fact, and as previously stated, ocular histoplasmosis instigates neovascularization of choroidal vessels, as can be noticed in **Figure 6**.

All in all, magnetic iron oxide nanoparticles can be a powerful strategy for cell-specific eye targeting. Their potential against *Candida* sp. has already been proven and amphotericin B has also been encapsulated in this nano system with enhanced fungicidal activity and reduced side effects [53]. In addition, these systems are biodegradable, intrinsically safe, exhibit increased half-life and their release localization can be controlled [52].

6. Vaccines for histoplasmosis

The creation of vaccination strategies for clinically relevant fungi has been a long-sought ambition for investigators, even with the difficulties assigned to these organisms' complex eukaryotic cells and their similarity to human proteins. Preventing or diminishing the severity of histoplasmosis through targeted vaccine development is then deemed to be an important scientific breakthrough [54, 55].

Glucan particles (GPs) are hollow, porous microspheres with an average diameter of 2–4 μm, derived from baker's yeast (*Saccharomyces cerevisiae*) purified cell walls and composed of 1,3-D-glucan and trace sums of chitin [56]. They are considered innovative and promising vaccine delivery systems, due to the possibility of encapsulating, transporting, delivering, and releasing protein antigens in their inner void cavity. In addition, the GPs delivery system retains the intrinsic immunostimulatory properties of 1,3-D-glucan on the surface. This polysaccharide functions as a ligand for receptor-mediated cell uptake by phagocytic cells bearing β-glucan receptors, for example, macrophages and dendritic cells in the immune system. Hence, GPs act as antigen-presenting phagocytic cells-selective-targeted delivery systems with adjuvant properties [55, 56].

A recent preclinical study was able to produce an extract from *H. capsulatum* yeast cells with the ability to convene protective immunity when encapsulated in GPs [21]. Succinctly, the GP vaccine consisted of *Histoplasma* alkaline extract, mouse serum albumin, and yeast RNA complexed with the glucan cells. Overall, the developed alkaline extract packaged in GP conferred vaccine-induced immunity, along with a reduced fungal burden by roughly 80% and improved survival in mice [56].

These data overlooks GP as useful vaccine delivery vehicles and may serve as a platform for the identification of proteins to include in GPs that both enhance protective immunity and modify immune responses to the agent [21]. On the other hand, this opens doors to the development of new GP nanoparticle-loaded formulations, which take advantage not only from the drug encapsulation assets of NPs but also from the macrophage-targeting properties of GPs [56].

Another ground-breaking study combining immunoproteomic and immunopeptidomic methods was able to map *H. capsulatum* peptide epitopes for the first time using murine dendritic cells and macrophages. After selecting and synthesizing the four most promising peptides, the incorporation into GPs took place. Efficient induction of $CD4^+$ and $CD8^+$ T lymphocytes was observed, as well as a production stimulation of IFN-γ, IL-17, and IL-2. The selected epitopes are derived from enolase (a heat shock protein 60) and the ATP-dependent molecular chaperone HSC82, which share a great degree of similarity with proteins expressed by other clinically relevant pathogenic fungi. Ergo, the authors preconize these promiscuous epitopes as the steppingstone for the creation of a multi-epitope peptide vaccine against histoplasmosis and other fungi [54].

7. Conclusion

Nanotechnology is still an emerging field in fungal vaccinology and pharmacology, yet there are many studies underlining its improved safety and tolerability. In fact, these innovative approaches have already replaced the original gold standard treatments for several forms of histoplasmosis disease, as outlined in this chapter.

Notwithstanding that, there are still a few therapeutic options to prevent and fight this neglected and potentially fatal disease. Therefore, the development of new drug delivery systems for the treatment and management of histoplasmosis is of utmost importance, particularly for AIDS patients.

Current investigation in antifungal drug delivery needs to put special emphasis on overcoming the challenges that deter the translation of nanoparticle-based systems into clinical practice.

Acknowledgements

This work was supported by the Foundation for Science and Technology, I.P. (FCT), Portugal, through grant reference 2020.05884.BD, and by the Applied Molecular Biosciences Unit – UCIBIO, which receives financial support from Portuguese national funds (FCT/MCTES, Fundação para a Ciência e Tecnologia and Ministério da Ciência, Tecnologia e Ensino Superior) through grant UIDB/04378/2020.

Conflict of interest

The authors declare no conflict of interest.

Author details

Filipa Sousa[1,2]*, Domingos Ferreira[1,2], Salette Reis[3] and Paulo Costa[1,2]

1 Faculty of Pharmacy, UCIBIO – Applied Molecular Biosciences Unit, MedTech-Laboratory of Pharmaceutical Technology, University of Porto, Portugal

2 Faculty of Pharmacy, Associate Laboratory i4HB - Institute for Health and Bioeconomy, University of Porto, Portugal

3 Faculty of Pharmacy, LAQV-REQUIMTE, Department of Chemical Sciences, University of Porto, Portugal

*Address all correspondence to: fsousa@ff.up.pt

References

[1] Azar MM, Loyd JL, Relich RF, Wheat LJ, Hage CA. Current concepts in the epidemiology, diagnosis, and Management of Histoplasmosis Syndromes. Seminars in Respiratory and Critical Care Medicine. 2020;**41**(1):13-30

[2] Kischkel B, Rossi SA, Santos SR, Nosanchuk JD, Travassos LR, Taborda CP. Therapies and vaccines based on nanoparticles for the treatment of systemic fungal infections. Frontiers in Cellular and Infection Microbiology. 2020;**10**:463

[3] Arauz AB, Papineni P. Histoplasmosis. Infectious Disease Clinics of North America. 2021;**35**(2):471-491

[4] Ashraf N, Kubat RC, Poplin V, Adenis AA, Denning DW, Wright L, et al. Re-drawing the maps for endemic mycoses. Mycopathologia. 2020;**185**(5):843-865

[5] Nacher M, Valdes A, Adenis A, Blaizot R, Abboud P, Demar M, et al. Disseminated histoplasmosis in HIV-infected patients: A description of 34 years of clinical and therapeutic practice. Journal of Fungi (Basel). 2020;**6**(3):164

[6] Guidelines for diagnosing and managing disseminated histoplasmosis among people living with HIV. 2020

[7] Purghè B, Manfredi M, Ragnoli B, Baldanzi G, Malerba M. Exosomes in chronic respiratory diseases. Biomedicine and Pharmacotherapy. 2021;**144**:112270

[8] Mejia SP, Lopez D, Cano LE, Naranjo TW, Orozco J. Antifungal encapsulated into ligand-functionalized nanoparticles with high specificity for macrophages. Pharmaceutics. 2022;**14**(9):1932

[9] Batista JM, Martins MAP, Bertollo CM. Primary cutaneous histoplasmosis difficult to treat in immunocompetent patient: Case report and literature review. Einstein (Sao Paulo). 2021;**19**:eRC5488

[10] Raina RK, Mahajan V, Sood A, Saurabh S. Primary cutaneous histoplasmosis in an immunocompetent host from a nonendemic area. Indian Journal of Dermatology. 2016;**61**(4):467

[11] Patra S, Nimitha P, Kaul S, Valakkada J, Verma K, Ramam M, et al. Primary cutaneous histoplasmosis in an immunocompetent patient presenting with severe pruritus. Indian Journal of Dermatology, Venereology and Leprology. 2018;**2018**:84

[12] Hariri OR, Minasian T, Quadri SA, Dyurgerova A, Farr S, Miulli DE, et al. Histoplasmosis with deep CNS involvement: Case presentation with discussion and literature review. Journal of Neurological Surgery Report. 2015;**76**(1):e167-e172

[13] Wheat J, Sarosi G, McKinsey D, Hamill R, Bradsher R, Johnson P, et al. Practice guidelines for the Management of Patients with histoplasmosis. Clinical Infectious Diseases. 2000;**30**(4):688-695

[14] Wheat LJ, Freifeld AG, Kleiman MB, Baddley JW, McKinscy DS, Loyd JE, et al. Clinical practice guidelines for the Management of Patients with histoplasmosis: 2007 update by the Infectious Diseases Society of America. Clinical Infectious Diseases. 2007;**45**(7):807-825

[15] Drak Alsibai K, Aissaoui H, Adenis A, Bourne-Watrin M, Djossou F, Epelboin L, et al. Cytological Spectrum of pulmonary histoplasmosis diagnosed by bronchoalveolar lavage: 12 years of

experience in French Guiana. Journal of Fungi (Basel). 2021;7(7):576

[16] Horwath MC, Fecher RA, Deepe GS Jr. Histoplasma capsulatum, lung infection and immunity. Future Microbiology. 2015;**10**(6):967-975

[17] Lamprecht A. Nanomedicines in gastroenterology and hepatology. Nature Reviews. Gastroenterology & Hepatology. 2015;**12**(4):195-204

[18] Dos Santos Ramos MA, Da Silva PB, Spósito L, De Toledo LG, Bonifácio BV, Rodero CF, et al. Nanotechnology-based drug delivery systems for control of microbial biofilms: A review. International Journal of Nanomedicine. 2018;**13**:1179-1213

[19] Pitangui NS, Sardi JC, Silva JF, Benaducci T, Moraes da Silva RA, Rodríguez-Arellanes G, et al. Adhesion of histoplasma capsulatum to pneumocytes and biofilm formation on an abiotic surface. Biofouling. 2012;**28**(7):711-718

[20] Suárez-Alvarez RO, Pérez-Torres A, Taylor ML. Adherence patterns of histoplasma capsulatum yeasts to bat tissue sections. Mycopathologia. 2010;**170**(2):79-87

[21] Deepe GS Jr, Buesing WR, Ostroff GR, Abraham A, Specht CA, Huang H, et al. Vaccination with an alkaline extract of histoplasma capsulatum packaged in glucan particles confers protective immunity in mice. Vaccine. 2018;**36**(23):3359-3367

[22] Sánchez A, Mejía SP, Orozco J. Recent advances in polymeric nanoparticle-encapsulated drugs against intracellular infections. Molecules. 2020;**25**(16):3670

[23] Mejia SP, Sanchez A, Vasquez V, Orozco J. Functional nanocarriers for delivering itraconazole against fungal intracellular infections. Frontiers in Pharmacology. 2021;**12**:685391

[24] Johnson PC, Wheat LJ, Cloud GA, Goldman M, Lancaster D, Bamberger DM, et al. Safety and efficacy of liposomal amphotericin B compared with conventional amphotericin B for induction therapy of histoplasmosis in patients with AIDS. Annals of Internal Medicine. 2002;**137**(2):105-109

[25] Fernández M, Orozco J. Advances in functionalized photosensitive polymeric nanocarriers. Polymers. 2021;**13**(15):2464

[26] Hay RJ. Liposomal amphotericin B, AmBisome. The Journal of infection. 1994;**28**(Suppl. 1):35-43

[27] Andrade F, Rafael D, Videira M, Ferreira D, Sosnik A, Sarmento B. Nanotechnology and pulmonary delivery to overcome resistance in infectious diseases. Advanced Drug Delivery Reviews. 2013;**65**(13-14):1816-1827

[28] Bressler NM, Bressler SB. Photodynamic therapy with verteporfin (Visudyne): Impact on ophthalmology and visual sciences. Investigative Ophthalmology & Visual Science. 2000;**41**(3):624-628

[29] Mônica Pereira Garcia MFMAS, Saldanha CA, RBA DCI. Amphotericin B: An antifungal drug in nanoformulations for the treatment of paracoccidioidomycosis. Revista de la Universidad Industrial de Santander Salud. 2013;**45**(3):45-53

[30] Cavassin FB, Baú-Carneiro JL, Vilas-Boas RR, Queiroz-Telles F. Sixty years of amphotericin B: An overview of the Main antifungal agent used to treat invasive fungal infections. Infectious Diseases and Therapy. 2021;**10**(1):115-147

[31] Saravolatz LD, Ostrosky-Zeichner L, Marr KA, Rex JH, Cohen SH.

Amphotericin B: Time for a new "gold standard". Clinical Infectious Diseases. 2003;**37**(3):415-425

[32] LeMonte AM, Washum KE, Smedema ML, Schnizlein-Bick C, Kohler SM, Wheat LJ. Amphotericin B combined with itraconazole or fluconazole for treatment of histoplasmosis. The Journal of Infectious Diseases. 2000;**182**(2):545-550

[33] Nagasa GD, Belete A. Review on nanomaterials and Nano-scaled Systems for Topical and Systemic Delivery of antifungal drugs. Journal of Multidisciplinary Healthcare. 2022;**15**:1819-1840

[34] Pilmis B, Jullien V, Sobel J, Lecuit M, Lortholary O, Charlier C. Antifungal drugs during pregnancy: An updated review. Journal of Antimicrobial Chemotherapy. 2014;**70**(1):14-22

[35] Wheat LJ, Cloud G, Johnson PC, Connolly P, Goldman M, Le Monte A, et al. Clearance of fungal burden during treatment of disseminated histoplasmosis with liposomal amphotericin B versus itraconazole. Antimicrobial Agents and Chemotherapy. 2001;**45**(8):2354-2357

[36] Garcia A, Adler-Moore JP, Proffitt RT. Single-dose AmBisome (Liposomal amphotericin B) as prophylaxis for murine systemic candidiasis and histoplasmosis. Antimicrobial Agents and Chemotherapy. 2000;**44**(9):2327-2332

[37] Santos G, Vasconcelos C, Lopes AJ, Cartágenes M, Barros Filho AK, Nascimento F, et al. Candida infections and therapeutic strategies: Mechanisms of action for traditional and alternative agents. Frontiers in Microbiology. 2018;**9**:1351

[38] Lim WM, Rajinikanth PS, Mallikarjun C, Kang YB. Formulation and delivery of itraconazole to the brain using a nanolipid carrier system. International Journal of Nanomedicine. 2014;**9**:2117-2126

[39] Sousa F, Ferreira D, Reis S, Costa P. Current insights on antifungal therapy: Novel nanotechnology approaches for drug delivery systems and new drugs from natural sources. Pharmaceuticals. 2020;**13**(9):248

[40] Mena-Giraldo P, Orozco J. Polymeric micro/nanocarriers and motors for cargo transport and phototriggered delivery. Polymers (Basel). 2021;**13**(22):3920

[41] Chen W, Zhan C, Gu B, Meng Q, Wang H, Lu W, et al. Targeted brain delivery of itraconazole via RVG29 anchored nanoparticles. Journal of Drug Targeting. 2011;**19**(3):228-234

[42] Beloqui A, Solinis MA, Rodriguez-Gascon A, Almeida AJ, Preat V. Nanostructured lipid carriers: Promising drug delivery systems for future clinics. Nanomedicine: Nanotechnology, Biology, and Medicine. 2016;**12**(1):143-161

[43] Ghosh S, Carter KA, Lovell JF. Liposomalformulationsofphotosensitizers. Biomaterials. 2019;**218**:119341

[44] Anselmo AC, Mitragotri S. Nanoparticles in the clinic: An update post COVID-19 vaccines. Bioengineering Translational Medicine. 2021;**6**(3):e10246

[45] Greco A, Garoffolo G, Chiesa E, Riva F, Dorati R, Modena T, et al. Nanotechnology, a booster for the multitarget drug verteporfin. Journal of Drug Delivery Science and Technology. 2021;**64**:102562

[46] Afarid M, Mahmoodi S, Baghban R. Recent achievements in nano-based technologies for ocular disease

diagnosis and treatment, review and update. Journal of Nanobiotechnology. 2022;**20**(1):361

[47] Ansar SM, Jiang W, Mudalige T. Analysis of verteporfin liposomal formulations for phospholipids and phospholipid degradation products by liquid chromatography-mass spectrometry (LC-MS). Journal of Pharmaceutical and Biomedical Analysis. 2022;**208**:114473

[48] Visudyne (verteporfin) [Summary of Product Characteristics]. European Medicines Agency, (Last update in September 2020). 2020

[49] de Oliveira DCS, de Freitas CF, Calori IR, Goncalves RS, Cardinali C, Malacarne LC, et al. Theranostic verteporfin- loaded lipid-polymer liposome for photodynamic applications. Journal of Photochemistry and Photobiology. B. 2020;**212**:112039

[50] Philip S, Kuriakose S. Synthesis, characterization and antimicrobial properties of superparamagnetic α-Fe2O3 nanoparticles stabilized by biocompatible starch. Journal of Cluster Science. 2021;**32**:1-11

[51] Philip S, Kuriakose S. Photodynamic antifungal activity of a superparamagnetic and fluorescent drug carrier system against antibiotic-resistant fungal strains. Cellulose (Lond). 2021;**28**(14):9091-9102

[52] Giannaccini M, Pedicini L, De Matienzo G, Chiellini F, Dente L, Raffa V. Magnetic nanoparticles: A strategy to target the choroidal layer in the posterior segment of the eye. Scientific Reports. 2017;**7**:43092

[53] Niemirowicz K, Durnaś B, Tokajuk G, Głuszek K, Wilczewska AZ, Misztalewska I, et al. Magnetic nanoparticles as a drug delivery system that enhance fungicidal activity of polyene antibiotics. Nanomedicine: Nanotechnology, Biology and Medicine. 2016;**12**(8):2395-2404

[54] Kischkel B, Boniche-Alfaro C, Menezes IG, Rossi SA, Angeli CB, de Almeida SR, et al. Immunoproteomic and Immunopeptidomic analyses of histoplasma capsulatum reveal promiscuous and conserved epitopes among Fungi with vaccine potential. Frontiers in Immunology. 2021;**12**:764501

[55] Mirza Z, Soto ER, Dikengil F, Levitz SM, Ostroff GR. Beta-Glucan Particles as Vaccine Adjuvant Carriers. Methods in Molecular Biology. 2017;**1625**:143-157

[56] Soto ER, Caras AC, Kut LC, Castle MK, Ostroff GR. Glucan particles for macrophage targeted delivery of nanoparticles. Journal of Drug Delivery. 2012;**2012**:143524

Chapter 8

HIV-Associated Histoplasmosis

Roxana-Carmen Cernat

Abstract

Impaired immunity induced by HIV is one of the main causes of disseminated histoplasmosis in endemic areas, and thus from 1987 WHO and then the CDC classified this condition as an AIDS-defining illness. Host factors associated independently with histoplasmosis are low level of CD4 (<150 cell/mm^3) and CD8 count, low nadir CD4, male gender, the absence of cART, the absence of systemic antifungals, and history of herpes simplex infection. Dissemination of an exogenously new acquired infection or reinfection and reactivation of a latent infection are both described in HIV-infected patients. Also, inflammatory reconstitution disease following cART initiation is possible. Acute pulmonary infection is rare, and only in HIV-infected patients with CD4 > 200 cell/mm^3. In advanced disease, the most frequent manifestation is as disseminated histoplasmosis often acute and severe, with complications such as respiratory failure, circulatory shock, and disseminated intravascular coagulation. The subacute presentation is frequent, associated with moderate involvement of the reticuloendothelial system, with great variability of clinical manifestation. Guidelines for diagnosing and managing histoplasmosis among people living with HIV have been published from WHO, IDSA, NIH, but limited data was based on randomized clinical trials.

Keywords: histoplasma capsulatum, immunocompromised patients, HIV, progressive disseminated histoplasmosis, impaired immunity

1. Introduction

Histoplasmosis as an endemic mycosis, overlapping the HIV pandemic, creates the most interesting and common pattern of infection in immunocompromised patients: the progressive disseminated form (PDF). Histoplasmosis is not a contagious disease, but in hyperendemic areas [1] (as regions of North America [2], Central America, and South America [3]), and also countries from Africa [4] and Asia [5] it has been reported to be the second or the third most common opportunistic infection in HIV-infected patients [6–9]; thus, this co-infection continues to generate clinical, diagnostic, and public health challenges. From 1987 histoplasmosis was classified by WHO as AIDS-defining disease, and from 2020 the same entity released guidelines for diagnosing and managing disseminated histoplasmosis among people living with HIV [1].

IntechOpen

2. Epidemiology

Histoplasmosis has been reported worldwide in tropical and subtropical, but most frequently, in temperate areas where this dimorphic fungus has found the perfect condition to thrive as mold (saprophytic form): nitrogen-rich soil at temperatures of 37°C or greater with moisture (95–100% humidity), containing bird droppings (composed of nutrients that promote growth and also substances that discourage the growth of competitive organisms), or bat guano.

However, what has significantly changed the global epidemiology of histoplasmosis was precisely the HIV pandemic, especially because of patients in the AIDS stage. In fact, HIV-infected patients often serve as sentinel markers for histoplasmosis outbreaks [6, 7].

Starting with 1983, several case reports have been published about HIV-infected patients who have been diagnosed with progressive disseminated histoplasmosis (PDH) [7]. Some of them came from endemic areas but a lot of cases have been discovered in places considered as non-endemic areas, which was not expected. In United States, reports have come from hyper-endemic areas such as Indiana [8, 9] as well as from areas where histoplasmosis has never been reported [10, 11] such as Denver or California.

Outside the United States, histoplasmosis incidence is driven by the AIDS pandemic [12]. In French Guyana, PDH is considered to be the most common AIDS-defining illness [12, 13], detected in 41% of HIV hospitalized patients with fever and CD4 less than 200 cell/mm^3. In the hyper-endemic area of Rio Grande do Sul, Brazil, 47% of patients diagnosed with histoplasmosis are HIV positive and have PDH [12, 14]. Between 1992 and 2008 in Columbia, 70.7% of the patient diagnosed with histoplasmosis had AIDS [12, 15, 16]. Two different studies estimated the incidence of histoplasmosis in Latin America to 1.48 cases per 100 PLWA, which amounts to over 22,000 cases per year [17, 18] (the first) and 0.15 per 100,000 person-years [18, 19] (the second), both estimation for 2012 and 2011. In the first study, countries with the highest histoplasmosis incidence in people living with HIV (≥1.5 cases per 100 people living with HIV) follow the same geographical distribution as histoplasmosis prevalence hotspots in the general population: Central America, Argentina, and the northernmost part of South America (Venezuela and the Guiana Shield) [17].

In parts of Asia [20], Southeast Asia [21], and India [22] where histoplasmosis is endemic, the most described and reported cases are in people living with HIV/AIDS. In China, 75% of cases are reported along the Yangtze River, most of them in association with AIDS [23].

In Africa, where HIV continues to be a major global public health issue [24], the estimated rate of histoplasmosis is not established due to the lack of solid epidemiologic studies and the limited possibility of detection in the laboratory. Cases of HIV patients have been reported in South Africa (Transvaal and Cape Province) [25], Zimbabwe [25], Uganda [26], Nigeria [27], and Tanzania [28]. Both strains of Histoplasma capsulatum are isolated in Africa. African histoplasmosis caused by H. capsulatum var. duboisii is prevalent in Western and Central Africa (Mali, Chad, Niger, Nigeria, Democratic Republic of Congo, and Ghana), and in the island of Madagascar [25]. Meanwhile, in South Africa and Zimbabwe, only the classical histoplasmosis caused by Histoplasma capsulatum var. capsulatum is known to occur [25] as is the case in the United States, Latin America, Asia, and Australia. Cases confirmed in HIV travelers who are returning home from these areas are diagnosed in Italy, Spain, the UK, the Netherlands, etc., as imported infections [29].

In Australia, where H. capsulatum has been found in Queensland and New South Wales from different samples (caves and fowl yards), only 63 cases have been diagnosed, but 41% of disseminated disease occurred in patients with human immunodeficiency virus [30].

In Europe, a non-endemic area, only a few cases of histoplasmosis in HIV-infected patients have been reported. Most of them are imported (mainly from Central and South America), but there were also rare autochthonous cases (Italy and Israel). The time span between leaving the endemic area and the diagnostic could reach up to four decades. Due to the scarce knowledge of this disease, the prognosis is poor with a high mortality rate (32%) [29] as the delay of diagnostic is detrimental in the course of disseminated histoplasmosis.

Due to the PDH form recognized by clinicians, reports about this disease came from across the world in places where histoplasmosis had been rarely or never present: Thailand, where this disease is observed almost exclusively among HIV-infected patients as this country is facing a high HIV prevalence (1253 cases reported from 1984 to 2010) [31, 32], Trinidad (only two cases also in HIV men) [33], and the Democratic Republic of Congo [18]. These reports of HIV patients are proving to be very useful in order to identify previously unrecognized areas where histoplasmosis could generate different forms of disease. Conversely, detecting a case of histoplasmosis in an area considered non-endemic must require the patient's testing for a possible HIV infection.

If prior to the advent of HAART approximately 5% of AIDS patients living in endemic area developed histoplasmosis [34] with a peak of incidence during the Indianapolis outbreak of 27% [6], nowadays initiating cART rapidly proves to be the game changer for this comorbidity in HIV patients [35, 36]. As the "test and treat" intervention strategy provides good results with 79% of people living with HIV aware of their status and 62% receiving treatment in 2018, and as guidelines recommend that all HIV-patient must start cART regardless of CD4 count [37–39], and it is expected that the global epidemiology of histoplasmosis in HIV patients will be changing in the future, except in countries where ART access is still not widely available or the patients are non-adherent.

Occupational risk factors identified to be associated with histoplasmosis in AIDS-patients were working with birds [35] or history of exposure to chicken coops [40]. Among case patients who had worked with soil contaminated with chicken or bat droppings and who could recall the date of their most recent exposure, the median time from their last exposure to the onset of symptoms was of 1.6 years [35]. A notable risk factor was smoking; although not historically associated with progressive disseminated histoplasmosis, smoking has been recognized as a risk factor for the chronic pulmonary form of the disease [41]. Recipients of antifungal agents as any triazole in the 2 months prior to the diagnosis of histoplasmosis seem to have a lower risk, as well as history of Pneumocystis jiroveci pneumonia (PCP) [35, 42].

Several risk factors are associated with the progressive disseminated form: low CD4 lymphocytes count (less than 150) and low nadir CD4 count [40, 42], low CD8 count [42], history of chronic medical condition and history of herpes simplex infection [35], and male gender [42]. Receiving treatment with TMP-SMZ was associated with a decreased risk of poor outcomes [35]. Other described factors associated with severe manifestations of histoplasmosis are: a level of creatinine higher than 2.1 mg/dL and hypoalbuminemia (less than 3/5 g/dL) [43].

3. Pathogenesis

Similar to other systemic fungal infections, the primary infection occurs in the lung after inhalation of the aerosolized microconidia. When the conidia reach the alveoli, the innate immune response is activated and the fungus binds to the CD11-CD18 family of integrins and is engulfed by neutrophils and macrophages [44, 45]. Once inhaled, the conidia transforms within hours into the parasitic yeast phase [18, 46]. Even though neutrophils emigrate early into infected foci of the lungs, these defense cells are fungistatic, not fungicidal, against Histoplasma capsulatum [47]. Macrophages and dendritic cells are the principal effector cells in host resistance to this fungus [44, 46], with a dual role in host defense for macrophages. H. capsulatum is able to replicate in macrophages until T cells will be activated, so the first role is to contain the yeast. The second role comes after cellular activation when several endogenous cytokines are released (IL-12, IFN-γ, TNF-α, and GM-CSF) and macrophages inhibit intracellular growth and harbor H. capsulatum, with granulomas formation [48, 49]. It is a protective mechanism to annihilate this fungus but also a repository for H. capsulatum that could lead to reactivation [48, 49]. Like tuberculosis, there is an early transport to regional lymph nodes with formation of a primary complex.

The link between innate and adaptive immunity is represented by dendritic cells that reside in the lung, as they are more potent than alveolar macrophages as antigen-presenting cells [50]. Dendritic cells have fungicidal activity and after phagocytosis will present H. capsulatum antigen to T cells, once they leave the tissues and travel to the lymph nodes. That generates the phase of adaptive immunity with lymphocyte proliferation and induction of cell-mediated immunity [51, 52]. T cells are crucial in clearance of H. capsulatum and this major implication is demonstrated by several experimental studies [53, 54]. Both CD4+ cells and CD8+ cells are necessary to induce a robust immune response [52, 55]. The adaptive immune response can either clear the organism of fungus or lead to granuloma formation. If the latter occurs, there is the potential for reactivation of the yeast. Reactivation is a response to impaired immunity. The primary contribution of T cells to host defense is the release of cytokines (IFN-γ, TNF-α, and GM-CSF) that will activate mononuclear phagocytes in order to control the infection.

HIV-infected patients are the perfect hosts for histoplasmosis especially in the late stage of AIDS. Depletion of CD4+ T cells and qualitative CD4+ T-cell dysfunction independent of T-cell depletion are the main mechanism that explains the increased susceptibility of these patients to opportunistic infections [56, 57]. Also, HIV decreases the circulating pool of effector and memory CD8+ T-cells that are able to combat viral infection with a final goal to enable CD8+ T-cell function [58]. In HIV patients, the depletion of T cells and their impaired activity are associated with lower level of cytokines such as IFN-γ and TNF-α that allow progressive disseminated histoplasmosis with increased fungal burden and mortality [44].

Macrophages resist HIV-1 infection much better than CD4+ T cells [59], but they have impaired activity against H. capsulatum [18, 44]. They bind fewer yeasts than cells from uninfected individuals as the HIV glycoprotein 120 envelope is responsible for this inhibition. A direct correlation is described between the CD4+ T-cell count and the capacity of macrophages to bind yeast cells. Once engulfed, yeasts grow more rapidly within macrophages from HIV-infected persons than in non-infected [44], and macrophages are not able to perform de second part of their defense in order to destroy H. capsulatum [60]. With a default immune response, macrophages cannot sterilize the infection, and dormant fungi from granuloma will be prone to reactivate.

The common histopathologic profile in HIV/AIDS co-infected patients with H. capsulatum is lack of organized inflammatory response with massive influx of macrophages and scarce number of lymphocytes. Thus, well-defined granulomas are infrequently present [61].

4. Clinical manifestations of H. capsulatum in HIV-infected patients

For primary histoplasmosis, the forms of disease depend on the degree of host immunosuppression and the yeast inoculum. Persons with higher CD4 + T-cell count, under cART, exposed to H. capsulatum could have no symptoms or develop an acute mild form of illness more often not recognized if the patients are not living in an endemic area. In this type of patients, the disease is restricted to the lungs as in general population but occurs in less than 5% of the cases [18]. On the opposite side, HIV-infected patients with scarce immunity (CD4 counts < 150 cells/mm^3) and not taking ART to develop progressive disseminated histoplasmosis. This is the most common profile of histoplasmosis, described in up to 95% of cases [62]. This pathway is common to exogenously acquired histoplasmosis as well as to reactivation and is determined by the hematogenous dissemination through the reticuloendothelial system (RES) that is containing parasitized macrophages. The term PDH describes the constant growth of organism in multiple organs rich in mononuclear phagocytes after the yeasts migrate from the lungs [45]. In endemic area, it is impossible to differentiate the reinfection to reactivation of dormant endogenous foci. Due to defective T-cell immunity in AIDS, reactivation seems to be the common pathway to histoplasmosis; however, autopsies series performed in the 1950s showed that although H. capsulatum is present in the lymph nodes, the cultures performed from these sites were sterile [45]. Thus, in endemic areas this evidence supports reinfection or progression of unrecognized histoplasmosis.

Depending on the degree involvement of RES and the underlying immune condition, different types of infection have been described. The acute disseminated form in AIDS patients is characterized by a high degree of RES involvement with closely packed macrophages engorged with yeast form [63] and have severe clinical implication as sepsis-like syndrome with septic shock, acute respiratory distress syndrome (ARDS), disseminated intravascular coagulation, neurological, hepatic, and renal involvement. Several cases of reactive hemophagocytic syndrome have been described [64] with bone marrow biopsy demonstrating the presence of histiocytes phagocytosing erythrocytes with poor outcome. Fever, weight loss, lymphadenopathy, hepatosplenomegaly, vomiting, and diarrhea are present as liver, spleen, bone marrow, and gastrointestinal tracts are the most commonly involved sites. Oropharyngeal and gastrointestinal mucosal ulcers are rarely present [63], but cutaneous lesions are described especially in Latin American late-diagnosed cases (66% versus up to 10% in the United States) [65]. The biopsy from cutaneous lesions (multiple disseminated papules, plaques, nodules, and pustules) could provide a simple and rapid diagnosis showing H. capsulatum yeasts intra- and extracellularly. CNS involvements such as encephalopathy, acute meningitis, or encephalitis are demonstrated in acute aggressive form of DPH with poor outcome [66]. Other atypical manifestations are described in acute form as chorioretinitis, colonic masses or anal ulcers, and pericarditis [45]. Acute disseminated forms rapidly evolve to death if untreated; therefore, rapid diagnosis and initiation of intravenous fungicidal therapy are required.

The second form of manifestation is subacute disseminated histoplasmosis, with a moderate involvement of the RES and also a moderate degree of macrophages parasitization [63]. Subacute or intermediate form is correlated with a longer interval of time when symptoms are present, in consequence a later presentation in the medical system. Manifestations are related to the development of focal lesions in various organs and associate with fever, weight loss, and weakness. Almost 25% of the patients have focal lesions in different organ systems, including gastrointestinal tract, endovascular, CNS, and adrenal glands [45, 63]. Gastrointestinal tract is commonly affected in subacute form, in addition to hepatic and splenic involvement. Lesions could be observed from the oropharynx to anus [67], but autopsies series demonstrate that the most affected parts are the colon and cecum followed by the terminal ileum with unique or multiple, deep, or diffuse ulcerations that lead to perforation or strictures, polypoid, and nodular masses that are complicated with obstruction. Symptoms frequently present in AIDS patients are: diarrhea, crampy abdominal pain, and tenderness in association with fever. Ascites, lower intestinal bleeding, and intestinal obstruction of the ileum are rare. In case of severe diarrhea, signs of malabsorption are present. Endoscopic examination especially of the right colon with subsequent biopsies could establish the diagnostic of PDH and exclude other AIDS-associated opportunistic infections (gastrointestinal tuberculosis and CVM colitis), cancers (Kaposi sarcoma and adenocarcinoma), idiopathic inflammatory bowel disease (ulcerative colitis and Crohn disease), and sarcoidosis. Systematic colonic biopsies must be performed in HIV-seropositive patients who have unexplained GI tract pathology because it can establish diagnosis in up to 89% of cases [68].

Endovascular forms of subacute PDH are represented by endocarditis on native or prosthetic valves, infection of abdominal aortic aneurysms, or prosthetic vascular grafts. These manifestations are rare, but in HIV patients who develop embolic phenomena in context of negative blood culture and extended vegetations on the left-sided valves (aortic valve), clinician must consider histoplasmosis.

Central nervous system (CNS) is involved in subacute PDH under several forms: subacute or chronic meningitis, diffuse encephalitis, cerebritis, focal granulomatosis lesions of the brain or spinal cord, and stroke due to fungi emboli [69, 70]. The CNS involvement in PDH is rare and the most common form is basal meningitis, even meningeal syndrome is described in less than 10% of these patients. Four classical forms of CNS histoplasmosis have been described, three of them in subacute form: isolated subacute or chronic meningitis, subacute or chronic form that associates other localizations (liver, lymphatic nodes, mucocutaneous, etc.), and focal lesions in the brain or histoplasmoma [71]. CNS symptoms during PDH have a slow progression starting with headache, confusion, and altered sensorium followed in weeks by seizures, ataxia, and focal deficits. Similar to tuberculosis, basilar meninges are affected, thus oculomotor nerves II, IV and VI are involved with cranial nerve palsy. In evolution, hydrocephalus could appear that requests neurosurgical evaluation for insertion of a shunt after few weeks of antifungal treatment [70]. The cerebrospinal fluid (CSF) is clear with pleocytosis (between 10 and 100 cells and the predominance of lymphocytes), elevated protein level, and hypoglycorrhachia in up to 80% of the patients. Direct examination of CSF is frequently negative, but culture could confirm histoplasmosis if the quantity and the time of growth are sufficient (several weeks are needed with the delay of the diagnosis). In subacute form of PDH in HIV-infected patients, due to the lack of antibodies in CSF correlated with the immunosuppression grade; this test is positive in less than 70% of the cases but Ag detection could provide a positive result in more than 90% of the cases [71]. Still, no technique is validated for detection of Histoplasma capsulatum antigen in CSF, this test being available only for urine samples. Histoplasmoma determines mass effect and the computer tomography scan detects ring enhancement with the administration of contrast, like in abscesses (toxoplasmosis) or malignancies [62]. The stereotactic brain biopsy is needed, and the result confirms the diagnosis as yeasts are detected in the caseous center of the granulomas [72].

Autopsy series have described others lesions as every single organ can be affected in subacute form of PDF. The involvement of adrenal glands has been reported in up to 80% of the cases although symptoms are rarely present and most of the time as unique manifestation [73]. At the gross examination, both adrenals are enlarged, which corresponded with the previously CT images performed. Focal areas containing parasitized macrophages can be found in both medulla and cortex. In severe infection, diffuse infiltration in parenchyma led to the destruction of both adrenal glands. Four categories of histopathological lesions have been described that are correlated with the host reaction against Histoplasma capsulatum: tuberculoid, anergic, mixed, and sequelae [74]. Adisson's disease with fever, malaise, nausea, vomiting, orthostatic hypotension, hyponatremia, and hyperkalemia occur in less than 10% of patients when extensive lesions have destroyed both adrenal glands.

Chronic progressive disseminated histoplasmosis is the third syndrome with the mildest RES involvement but also with the mildest macrophages parasitization [63], and is characterized by mildest and prolonged manifestation during years, occasionally intermittent and it is described only in adult people. Constitutional symptoms such as fatigue, weakness, gradual weight loss, malaise, lethargy, and low-grade fever are intermittently present. The pathognomonic sign is oropharyngeal ulcerations that are well delimited, deep, and painless. All the mucosal areas could be involved: oral cavity, lips, tongue, pharynx, nasal septum, larynx, labia, or penis. Biopsies performed for single lesions to exclude oral squamous carcinoma indicate granulomas with macrophages containing yeasts, but simple MGG-stained smears (May-Grunwald-Giemsa) or periodic acid-Schiff stains are useful to visualize Histoplasma capsulatum. Hepatosplenomegaly is present in almost a third of the patients, and in few cases, chronic granulomatous hepatitis has been described [75]. Chronic meningitis appears as single manifestation of the disease [45], in contrast to the subacute form where multiple organs are involved. Endocarditis, bone infection (septic arthritis and osteomyelitis), Addison disease, and pancytopenia caused by bone marrow suppression have been cited in literature as uncommon. Not recognized and treated, chronic PDH progresses to death.

Another distinct form is immune reconstitution inflammatory syndrome (IRIS) as a complication of starting cART in HIV-infected patients when a decay greater than 1 log in viral load associates inflammatory and atypical clinical features with signs and symptoms unexplained by a newly acquired infection or treatment failure [75, 76]. Both forms have been described as the immune system begins to recover following treatment: "unmasking" IRIS (flare-up of an underlying and previously undiagnosed histoplasmosis) and "paradoxical" IRIS (flare-up of a previously treated histoplasmosis). Compared to other pathogens, the incidence of histoplasmosis-associated IRIS is low (0.74 cases at 1000 HIV-infected person-years) and remain stable during the last 20 years in French Guyana where histoplasmosis is the most frequent opportunistic infection in HIV [76]. The clinical findings are polymorphic as in disseminated form with fever, lymph node enlargement, digestive, hematologic, respiratory, mucocutaneous manifestations and less frequent neurological, rheumatological, or ocular involvement [76].

Some clinical differences have been noted between the two variants, especially in Africa where H. capsulatum var. capsulatum coexists with H. capsulatum var. duboisii and HIV-epidemic remain the main health problem in the last decades. Due to the tropism of the variety duboisii for lymph nodes, skin, and bones, in HIV-infected patients, the dissemination of this yeast associates with classical PDH ulcers, nodules, psoriasis plaque, subcutaneous nodules, osteolytic lesions in the skull, ribs, vertebrae and enlarged lymph nodes [4].

Co-infections with other opportunistic infections have been described, due to the immunocompromised status of HIV-infected patients. In countries from Latin-America, the percentage of triple infections is very high: Columbia (51%), Brazil (43%), Argentina (42%), French Guyana (37–42%), and Panama (25%) [77].

The most reported is association with tuberculosis as this is the leading opportunistic infection related to HIV [77–80]. Both are able to spread and determine miliary forms and granuloma formation. The overlapping symptoms can delay the final and complete diagnosis. In this context, constitutional signs are frequently present with respiratory symptoms in only half of the patients despite that chest X-rays reveal infiltrates of the lungs [78]. Other common clinical findings associated with fever are: lymphadenopathy, hepatomegaly, splenomegaly, gastrointestinal pain, abnormal liver function tests, anemia, leukopenia, and thrombocytopenia [79]. If tuberculosis diagnosis is rapid by direct microscopic observation of acid-fast-bacilli (AFB), the histoplasmosis diagnosis confirmation is more difficult, primarily by histopathology if the patient is not living in an endemic area. Blood and bone marrow culture are useful to diagnose both disseminated diseases [79]. Co-occurrence of TB/histoplasmosis disseminated infections must be suspected by the persistence of the symptoms after completion of anti-Koch's regimen in patients with confirmed TB; thus, H. capsulatum must be tested from different specimens [80].

Other opportunistic infections (OI's) associated with histoplasmosis-HIV coinfection have been described: pneumocystosis [81], cryptococcal infection [82], cytomegalovirus infection, Salmonella infection, candidiasis, and toxoplasmosis [75]. Sometimes, more co-infections could be hosted by the same HIV-infected person [83]. As all of them are associated with severe immunodepression and have non-specific clinical signs and symptoms, clinicians must by aware of these possibilities and investigate in order to confirm the diagnostic and to provide appropriate treatment.

5. Diagnosis

In non-endemic areas where clinicians and pathologists are not aware of this pathology, the diagnostic of histoplasmosis in HIV-infected patients is difficult due to the unspecific symptoms in progressive disseminated form. For clinicians, it is important to remember that even short exposure in endemic area should be a reason to consider histoplasmosis in HIV-infected patients, as early and rapid diagnosis followed by initiation of optimal treatment is able to improve survival.

In April 2020, WHO released a set of recommendations for the management of histoplasmosis among PLWHIV [1], which contain guidelines for the diagnosis and treatment with the aim to provide the same approach for the entire health system, not only for the countries that face the highest burden as North America, Central America, South America, and some countries from Asia and Africa.

According these guidelines, "test and treat" concept for detecting and treating all HIV-infected persons is the most important strategy as this reduce the number of opportunistic infections, including histoplasmosis. Further, among people living with HIV, "disseminated histoplasmosis should be diagnosed by detecting circulating Histoplasma antigen" on the basis that:

- Traditional gold standard (culture from peripheral blood or tissue specimens, histopathologic analysis, and special stains) is based on conventional laboratory tests that have their limitations in terms of time and performance, imposing Biosafety Level 3 Laboratory infrastructures with trained personnel;

- Serodiagnosis tests that detect the presence of antibodies against Histoplasma capsulatum have decreased sensibility in immunosuppressed patients and are not able to differentiate the active from past infection; also, they cross-react with other antigens from Coccidioides, Paracoccidioides, or Blastomyces;

- Molecular testing of DNA detection has high accuracy but there is a lack of consensus, technique, and availability of kits;

- Antigen detection assays are the most accurate to diagnose progressive disseminated histoplasmosis in HIV-infected persons. These tests are available, affordable, and can be performed in all laboratories (Biosafety Level 1 and 2) from non-invasive samples (urine) and reduce the time to diagnosis.

Urine antigen detection test is more sensitive than the serum antigen test for AIDS patients with disseminated histoplasmosis. Different publications showed that 92–100% of patients have antigenuria compared to almost 50–92.3% who present antigenemia [64, 84] depending on the type of assay. False-positive results in testing urinary antigen assay could appear in other mycoses as Blastomyces dermatitidis, Talaromyces marneffey, and Paracoccidioides brasiliensis because they have the same class of cell wall galactomannan, but not in aspergillosis [84]. In transplant recipients who received thymoglobulin or in cases associated with the presence of rheumatoid factor, the Histoplasma serum antigen could be false positive, and thus, urinary Ag is required [64].

Antigen detection is an important tool for monitoring the therapeutic response. In case of persistent antigenuria with failure to decrease after 1 month of treatment an ongoing infection is present [85]; meanwhile, increased titers should advise about the possibility of relapse [86]. For CNS histoplasmosis, antigen detection is a reliable to orientate the diagnosis as this becomes positive in less than one week combined with detection of antibodies from CSF and serum, as culture requires more than 2 weeks for growth [87].

However, the investigation of an HIV-infected person must be comprehensive, in order to evaluate the immune status of the patient and the extension of the disease. Also, other co-infection must be ruled out. Some unspecific biological abnormalities could indicate PDH as adjunct laboratory markers: very high level of serum lactate dehydrogenase (>600 UI/ml) [88], increased level of ferritin (>1000 ng/ml) [45, 89], increased AST level associated with increased alkaline phosphate and thrombocytopenia [88, 90], and hematuria and proteinuria [90].

6. Treatment

Patients with CD4 count > 300 cells/mm^3 who develop acute pulmonary histoplasmosis must be treated as immunocompetent persons [91].

Progressive disseminated histoplasmosis in HIV-infected patients is a life-threatening infection that requires always treatment, as the mortality rate in untreated infection is very high (up to 100%) [91].

Several guidelines have been released with recommendations for treatment for disseminated form of histoplasmosis in people living with HIV: IDSA, DHHS, EACS, WHO. According to the last one published in 2020, the treatment is related to the form of the infection considering that:

-Severe and moderate-severe form is defined as the presence of at least one symptom or sign that involved vital organs and with a general alteration of WHO performance status more than 2; mild and mild-to-moderate form have no symptoms or signs listed before;

-cART should be initiated as soon as possible if histoplasmosis CNS involvement is not suspected or proven as this poses additional challenges and requires different approach than the other forms [1].

The preferred regimen for severe or moderate-severe form as induction therapy is intravenous liposomal amphotericin B (3 mg/kg/day) for up to two weeks, as this formulation has demonstrated better outcomes than standard deoxycholate formulation in terms of rapid and complete response (82% versus 56%), lower mortality (2% versus 13%), and nephrotoxicity (9% versus 37%) [92]. Clinical improvement (resolution of fever and no need for ventilatory support, or vasopressors) must be followed by step-down therapy to itraconazole 200 mg three times a day for 3 days, and then 200 mg twice a day for at least 12 months as maintenance treatment [1, 91, 93].

If liposomal formulation is not available, standard deoxycholate amphotericin B must be initiated in dose of 0.7–1.0 mg/kg/day with close monitoring of the renal function and electrolytes. Dose reduction or rapid switch to itraconazole is needed if the patient develops nephrotoxicity despite proactive fluids and electrolytes replacement or other toxicities (anemia and toxic-related infusion).

Intravenous amphotericin B lipid complex at 5 mg/kg/day is an alternative option but it demonstrated a lower efficacy than two previous options [18] in AIDS patients with PDH.

Itraconazole is preferred for induction and maintenance therapy for mild or mild to moderate forms of histoplasmosis in HIV-infected patients. After 3 days of 200 mg three times a day as loading dose, 200 mg twice a day must be continued for at least 12 months, with dose adjustment based on drug-drug interaction with ARV and itraconazole serum concentration [1, 91, 93]. Itraconazole must be administrated with food or low-pH beverages (such as cola) in order to increase absorption. Liquid itraconazole is preferred due to better absorption if it is well tolerated. Blood level must be measured after 2 weeks of treatment (time to reach steady state) to verify if achieving optimal concentration between 1 and 2 mcg/ml. Serum concentrations could be useful in case of drug-drug interactions or to assess the adherence of the patient. Higher concentration (>15 mcg/ml) is correlated with toxicities. Most adverse events in HIV-infected patients are nausea, vomiting, rash, and pedal edema.

Like all the triazoles, itraconazole exhibits multiple drug interactions, most notably with cytochrome P450-inducing drugs [94]. Before starting treatment, these potential drug-drug interactions must be evaluated as HIV infection must be treated as well. Non-nucleoside reverse transcriptase inhibitors (NNRTIs) such as Efavirenz (EFV), Nevirapine (NVP), and Etravirine (ETR) reduce itraconazole blood level; meanwhile, Doravirine (DOR) display only low interactions and co-administration does not require TDM for itraconazole like for previous ones. Boosted protease inhibitors (PIs) such as lopinavir (LPV/r), atazanavir (ATZ/r), darunavir (DRV/r or DRV/c) increase itraconazole blood level so must be avoided or TDM is needed to avoid toxicities. Integrase inhibitors (INSTI) such as Raltegravir or Dolutegravir have no interaction so are safe to prescribe them in association with itraconazole but, due to cobicistat, Elvitegravir will increase itraconazole level [95] and must be avoided. Tuberculosis medication's rifampicin and rifabutin, potent inducers of cytochrome P450 (CYP) enzymes and transporters, decrease the level of itraconazole; on the other hand, itraconazole may increase the blood levels of rifabutin [94, 95].

If itraconazole cannot be administrated, alternative therapy must be considered for treating less severe disseminated disease. Posaconazole is the preferred antifungal for treating H. capsulatum as it demonstrates high efficacy in patients who failed other fungicidal medication [96]. Posaconazole treatment duration ranged from 6 weeks to 48 weeks depending on the clinical form and was followed by successful clinical outcomes [97]. Serum level must be measured after 5 days in order to reach steady state to determine if the drug has adequate absorption (concentration must be >1 mcg/mL). Fluconazole 800 mg once daily is associated with a slower decline of antigenuria than itraconazole [98] and with a higher rate of resistance emergence in HIV-infected patients due to a single point mutation [99], so is no longer recommended as maintenance therapy [100]. Voriconazole was associated with increased mortality in the first 42 days when compared to itraconazole in a retrospective cohort in which have been included 24.7% HIV-infected patients with disseminated histoplasmosis [101]. Isavuconazole could be an alternative to Posaconazole and cases have been published with good outcome [102], but there are not enough data to generate a conclusion.

The maintenance therapy with itraconazole in AIDS-associated disseminated histoplasmosis must be 12 months in order to suppress residual infection and to prevent relapses. Is safe to discontinue itraconazole after 12 months when CNS involvement is absent, CD4 counts are more than 150 cells/mm^3, HIV-RNA is suppressed under cART, and Histoplasma antigenuria is less than 2 ng/mL [35], otherwise must be continued with 200 mg/day for the entire life as long-term suppressive therapy [91, 93]. In some cases, itraconazole can be replaced by Posaconazole XR 300 mg/day (best option), Fluconazole 400 mg/day, or Voriconazole 200 mg/day.

A special approach must be considered for H. capsulatum meningitis. The induction therapy with intravenous liposomal amphotericin B 5 mg/kg/day must be longer, for 4–6 weeks, followed by itraconazole 200 mg two or three times a day for more than 12 months with dosage adjusted not to exceed 10 mcg/mL [91, 93]. The maintenance treatment with Itraconazole must be continued till the resolution of CNS abnormal findings with negative antigen and culture of CSF when CD4 count recovered as HIV viral load became undetectable. Itraconazole could be replaced in case of intolerance by Posaconazole as alternative best option, Fluconazole, or Voriconazole.

All guidelines recommend monitoring treatment response by performing antigen level at the initiation of antifungal medication; at the end of amphotericin B induction phase, at 3, 6, and 12 months and when it is decided the cessation of therapy [1, 91, 93]. Any increase in antigen level must be followed by a comprehensive evaluation considering adherence to antifungal and ARV treatment. TDM for itraconazole level is required, and also CD4 count and HIV-RNA determination as relapses are related to non-adherence [35].

Antiretroviral therapy should be initiated as soon as possible if CNS involvement is not suspected or confirmed [1, 91]. In order to avoid drug-drug interaction with any triazole, INSTI-based regimen (DTG or RAL) are preferred as first-line therapy or doravirine (DOR) as NNRTI-based regimen. Immune reconstitution inflammatory syndrome (IRIS) is uncommon in HIV-infected people with histoplasmosis with an incidence rate of 0.74 cases/1000 HIV-infected person-years [76]; thus, the cART should not be delayed. The management of IRIS associated with histoplasmosis is to continue antiretroviral treatment as well as antifungal therapy with short term of oral steroids associated (Prednison 1 mg/kg per day) if there are life-threatening complications. If patient is naïve to cART, a two-week delay is recommended before starting medication; meanwhile, induction antifungal therapy is in place.

The most challenging situation for clinicians is treatment of histoplasmosis/tuberculosis co-occurrence in HIV-infected patients as currently, there are no guidelines or recommendations targeting all three infections. Tuberculosis must be treated according WHO, DHHS, EACS guidelines, but due to drug-drug interactions, especially in HIV heavily pretreated patients requiring protease inhibitors regimens or in case of MDR-tuberculosis, clinicians must seek experts advise. Due to drug-drug interactions between itraconazole—rifampin or rifabutin—some ARV drugs, TDM for itraconazole must be perform on a regular basis. Results from a case series study conducted in Columbia on 12 PLHIV determined investigators to recommend fluoroquinolone instead of rifampicin use for TB as three patients treated with rifampicin had undetectable levels of itraconazole [78]. Another challenge is delaying initiation of ARV therapy up to 14 days as CD4 count is frequent less than 200 cells/mm^3, due to the associated risk of developing IRIS [76].

7. Preventing exposure

HIV-infected persons with CD4 count <150 cells/mm^3 should avoid activities associated with high risk for histoplasmosis: cleaning chicken coops, disturbing area contaminate with bird or bat droppings, exploring caves, demolishing old buildings, and creating dust as they are working with surface soil [91, 93].

8. Primary prophylaxis

In high endemic areas (incidence >10 cases/100 patients-years), primary prophylaxis with Itraconazole 200 mg daily in HIV-infected patients with severe immunodepression reduce the frequency but not the mortality due to histoplasmosis [103], and thus is recommended for patients with CD4 count <150 cells/mm with high risk due to occupational exposure. The primary prophylaxis must be discontinued if the immune status is improving when CD4 counts attaint 150 cells/mm^3 and remain stable for more than 6 months, and must be restarted when CD4 count decreases <150 cells/mm [93].

9. Conclusions

Histoplasmosis overlapping HIV-pandemic redefined the epidemiology and the clinical features of this disease, generating a particular form in AIDS: progressive disseminated histoplasmosis. Challenges in diagnosis (especially in non-endemic areas where a significant knowledge gap still exists), treatment (due to drug-drug interactions between fungicidal drugs and cART, and availability of medications) and association with other opportunistic infections (especially tuberculosis) have determined specialists to release guidelines but also research priorities. Hopefully, access to antiretroviral medication for all HIV patients will change the face of this pathology till new strategies will be available in order to control this potentially life-threatening illness.

Author details

Roxana-Carmen Cernat
Clinical Hospital of Infectious Diseases, "Ovidius" University Constanta, Romania

*Address all correspondence to: roxana.cernat@365.univ-ovidius.ro

References

[1] WHO. Guidelines for Diagnosing and Managing Disseminated Histoplasmosis among People Living with HIV. Washington, DC: Pan American Health Organization, and Geneva: World Health Organization; Apr 2020

[2] Manos NE, Ferebee SH, Kerschbaum WF. Geographic variation in the prevalence of histoplasmin sensitivity. Dis Chest. 1956;**29**(6):649-668. DOI: 10.1378/chest.29.6.649

[3] Colombo AL, Tobón A, Restrepo A, Queiroz-Telles F, Nucci M. Epidemiology of endemic systemic fungal infections in Latin America. Med Mycol. 2011;**49**(8):785-798. DOI: 10.3109/13693786.2011.577821 Epub 2011 May 4

[4] Loulergue P, Bastides F, Baudouin V, Chandenier J, Mariani-Kurkdjian P, Dupont B, et al. Literature review and case histories of Histoplasma capsulatum var. duboisii infections in HIV-infected patients. Emerg Infect Dis. 2007;**13**(11):1647-1652. DOI: 10.3201/eid1311.070665

[5] Chakrabarti A, Slavin MA. Endemic fungal infections in the Asia-Pacific region. Med Mycol. 2011;**49**(4):337-344. DOI: 10.3109/13693786.2010.551426 Epub 2011 Jan 24

[6] Wheat LJ, Connolly-Stringfield PA, Baker RL, Curfman MF, Eads ME, Israel KS, et al. Disseminated histoplasmosis in the acquired immune deficiency syndrome: Clinical findings, diagnosis and treatment, and review of the literature. Medicine (Baltimore). 1990;**69**(6):361-374. DOI: 10.1097/00005792-199011000-00004

[7] Bahr NC, Antinori S, Wheat LJ, Sarosi GA. Histoplasmosis infections worldwide: Thinking outside of the Ohio River valley. Curr Trop Med Rep. 2015;**2**(2):70-80. DOI: 10.1007/s40475-015-0044-0

[8] Sathapatayavongs B, Batteiger BE, Wheat J, Slama TG, Wass JL. Clinical and laboratory features of disseminated histoplasmosis during two large urban outbreaks. Medicine (Baltimore). 1983;**62**(5):263-270. DOI:10.1097/00005792-198309000-00001

[9] Wheat LJ, Slama TG, Zeckel ML. Histoplasmosis in the acquired immune deficiency syndrome. Am J Med. 1985;**78**(2):203-210. DOI: 10.1016/0002-9343(85)90427-9

[10] Kaur J, Myers AM. Homosexuality, steroid therapy, and histoplasmosis. Ann Intern Med. 1983;**99**(4):567. DOI: 10.7326/0003-4819-99-4-567_1

[11] Haggerty CM, Britton MC, Dorman JM, Marzoni FA Jr. Gastrointestinal histoplasmosis in suspected acquired immunodeficiency syndrome. West J Med. 1985;**143**(2):244-246

[12] Wheat LJ, Azar MM, Bahr NC, Spec A, Relich RF, Hage C. Histoplasmosis. Infect Dis Clin North Am. 2016;**30**(1):207-227. DOI: 10.1016/j.idc.2015.10.009

[13] Epelboin L, Dione A, Serris A, Blanchet D, Bidaud B, Walter G, et al. Histoplasmosis of the central nervous system: A case series between 1990 and 2019 in French Guiana. Am J Trop Med Hyg. 2021;**105**(1):125-129. DOI: 10.4269/ajtmh.20-1486

[14] Severo LC, de Oliveira FM, Irion K, da Porto NS, Londero AT. Histoplasmosis

in Rio Grande do Sul, Brazil: A 21-year experience. Rev Inst Med trop S Paulo. 2001;**43**(4):183-187. DOI: 10.1590/S0036-46652001000400001

[15] Arango M, Castañeda E, Agudelo CI, De Bedout C, Agudelo CA, Tobón A, et al. Histoplasmosis: Results of the Colombian national survey, 1992-2008. Biomedica. 2011;**31**(3):344-356. DOI: 10.1590/S0120-41572011000300007

[16] Adenis AA, Valdes A, Cropet C, McCotter OZ, Derado G, Couppie P, et al. Burden of HIV-associated histoplasmosis compared with tuberculosis in Latin America: A modelling study. Lancet Infect Dis. 2018;**18**(10):1150-1159. DOI: 10.1016/S1473-3099(18)30354-2 Epub 2018 Aug 23

[17] Myint T, Leedy N, Villacorta Cari E, Wheat LJ. HIV-associated histoplasmosis: Current perspectives. HIV AIDS (Auckl). 2020;**12**:113-125. DOI: 10.2147/HIV.S185631

[18] Nacher M, Adenis A, Adriouch L, Dufour J, Papot E, Hanf M, et al. What is AIDS in the Amazon and the Guianas? Establishing the burden of disseminated histoplasmosis. Am J Trop Med Hyg. 2011;**84**(2):239-240. DOI: 10.4269/ajtmh.2011.10-0251

[19] Randhawa HS. Occurrence of histoplasmosis in Asia. Mycopathol Mycol Appl. 1970;**41**(1):75-89. DOI: 10.1007/BF02051485

[20] Baker J, Setianingrum F, Wahyuningsih R, Denning DW. Mapping histoplasmosis in South East Asia - implications for diagnosis in AIDS. Emerg Microbes Infect. 2019;**8**(1):1139-1145. DOI: 10.1080/22221751.2019.1644539

[21] Randhawa HS, Gugnan HC. Occurrence of histoplasmosis in the Indian sub-continent: An overview and update. Journal of Medical Research and Practice. 2018;**7**:71-83

[22] Pan B, Chen M, Pan W, Liao W. Histoplasmosis: A new endemic fungal infection in China? Review and analysis of cases. Mycoses. 2013;**56**(3):212-221. DOI: 10.1111/myc.12029 Epub 2012 Dec 10

[23] WHO Regional Office for Africa. Preventing and Responding to HIV Drug Resistance in the African Region: Regional Action Plan 2019-2023. ISBN: 978-929023422-7

[24] Gugnani HC. Histoplasmosis in Africa: A review. Indian J Chest Dis Allied Sci. 2000;**42**:271-277

[25] Bahr NC, Sarosi GA, Meya DB, Bohjanen PR, Richer SM, Swartzentruber S, et al. Seroprevalence of histoplasmosis in Kampala, Uganda. Med Mycol. 2016;**54**(3):295-300. DOI: 10.1093/mmy/myv081 Epub 2015 Nov 2

[26] Oladele RO, Toriello C, Ogunsola FT, Ayanlowo OO, Foden P, Fayemiwo AS, et al. Prior subclinical histoplasmosis revealed in Nigeria using histoplasmin skin testing. PLoS One. 2018;**13**(5):e0196224. DOI: 10.1371/journal.pone.0196224

[27] Lofgren SM, Kirsch EJ, Maro VP, Morrissey AB, Msuya LJ, Kinabo GD, et al. Histoplasmosis among hospitalized febrile patients in northern Tanzania. Trans R Soc Trop Med Hyg. 2012;**106**(8):504-507. DOI: 10.1016/j.trstmh.2012.05.009 Epub 2012 Jun 26

[28] Antinori S, Giacomelli A, Corbellino M, Torre A, Schiuma M, Casalini G, et al. Histoplasmosis diagnosed in Europe and Israel: A case report and systematic review of the literature from 2005 to 2020. J Fungi (Basel). 2021;7(6):481. DOI: 10.3390/jof7060481

[29] McLeod DSA, Mortimer RH, Perry-Keene DA, Allworth A, Woods ML, Perry-Keene J, et al. Histoplasmosis in Australia: Report of 16 cases and literature review. Medicine (Baltimore). 2011;**90**(1):61-68. DOI: 10.1097/MD.0b013e318206e499

[30] Antinori S. Histoplasma capsulatum: More widespread than previously thought. Am J Trop Med Hyg. 2014;**90**(6):982-983. DOI: 10.4269/ajtmh.14-0175 Epub 2014 Apr 28

[31] Norkaew T, Ohno H, Sriburee P, Tanabe K, Tharavichitkul P, Takarn P, et al. Detection of environmental sources of Histoplasma capsulatum in Chiang Mai, Thailand, by nested PCR. Mycopathologia. 2013;**176**(5-6):395-402. DOI: 10.1007/s11046-013-9701-9 Epub 2013 Sep 13

[32] Bartholomew C, Raju C, Patrick A, Penco F, Jankey N. AIDS on Trinidad. Lancet. 1984;**1**(8368):103. DOI: 10.1016/s0140-6736(84)90029-1

[33] Hajjeh RA. Disseminated histoplasmosis in persons infected with human immunodeficiency virus. Clin Infect Dis. 1995;**21**(Suppl 1):S108-S110. DOI: 10.1093/clinids/21.supplement_1.s108

[34] Hajjeh RA, Pappas PG, Henderson H, Lancaster D, Bamberger DM, Skahan KJ, et al. Multicenter case-control study of risk factors for histoplasmosis in human immunodeficiency virus-infected persons. Clin Infect Dis. 2001;**32**(8):1215-1220. DOI: 10.1086/319756 Epub 2001 Mar 26

[35] Myint T, Anderson AM, Sanchez A, Farabi A, Hage C, Baddley JW, et al. Histoplasmosis in patients with human immunodeficiency virus/acquired immunodeficiency syndrome (HIV/AIDS): Multicenter study of outcomes and factors associated with relapse. Medicine (Baltimore). 2014;**93**(1):11-18. DOI: 10.1097/MD.0000000000000016

[36] World Health Organization. Consolidated Guidelines on HIV, Viral Hepatitis and STI Prevention, Diagnosis, Treatment, and Care for Key Populations. WHO; 2022

[37] Panel on Antiretroviral Guidelines for Adults and Adolescents. Guidelines for the Use of Antiretroviral Agents in Adults and Adolescents with HIV. Department of Health and Human Services;

[38] European AIDS Clinical Society EACS Guidelines, version 11.1. 2022. Available from: https://www.eacsociety.org/media/guidelines-11.1_final_09-10.pdf

[39] McKinsey DS, Spiegel RA, Hutwagner L, Stanford J, Driks MR, Brewer J, et al. Prospective study of histoplasmosis in patients infected with human immunodeficiency virus: Incidence, risk factors, and pathophysiology. Clin Infect Dis. 1997;**24**(6):1195-1203. DOI: 10.1086/513653

[40] Oladele RO, Osaigbovo II, Akanmu AS, Adekanmbi OA, Ekeng BE, Mohammed Y, et al. Prevalence of histoplasmosis among persons with advanced HIV disease. Nigeria. Emerg Infect Dis. 2022;**28**(11):2261-2269. DOI: 10.3201/eid2811.220542

[41] Nacher M, Adenis A, Blanchet D, Vantilcke V, Demar M, Basurko C, et al. Risk factors for disseminated histoplasmosis in a cohort of HIV-infected patients in French Guiana. PLoS Negl Trop Dis. 2014;**8**(1):e2638. DOI: 10.1371/journal.pntd.0002638

[42] Wheat LJ, Chetchotisakd P, Williams B, Connolly P, Shutt K, Hajjeh R. Factors associated with severe manifestations of histoplasmosis in AIDS. Clin Infect Dis. 2000;**30**(6):877-881. DOI: 10.1086/313824 Epub 2000 Jun 14

[43] Newman SL. Macrophages in host defense against Histoplasma capsulatum.

Trends Microbiol. 1999;**7**(2):67-71. DOI: 10.1016/s0966-842x(98)01431-0

[44] Deepe GS Jr. Histoplasma capsulatum (histoplasmosis). In: Mandell, Douglas, and Bennett's Principles and Practice of Infectious Diseases. 9th ed. Elsevier; 2020. pp. 3162-3176

[45] Woods JP, Heinecke EL, Luecke JW, Maldonado E, Ng JZ, Retallack DM, et al. Pathogenesis of Histoplasma capsulatum. Semin Respir Infect. 2001;**16**(2):91-101. DOI: 10.1053/srin.2001.24239

[46] Newman SL, Gootee L, Gabay JE, Selsted ME. Identification of constituents of human neutrophil azurophil granules that mediate fungistasis against Histoplasma capsulatum. Infect Immun. 2000;**68**(10):5668-5672. DOI: 10.1128/IAI.68.10.5668-5672.2000

[47] Deepe GS Jr, Gibbons RS, Smulian AG. Histoplasma capsulatum manifests preferential invasion of phagocytic subpopulations in murine lungs. J Leukoc Biol. 2008;**84**(3):669-678. DOI: 10.1189/jlb.0308154 Epub 2008 Jun 24

[48] Horwath MC, Fecher RA, Deepe GS Jr. Histoplasma capsulatum, lung infection and immunity. Future Microbiol. 2015;**10**:967-975. DOI: 10.2217/fmb.15.25

[49] Gildea LA, Morris RE, Newman SL. Histoplasma capsulatum yeasts are phagocytosed via very late antigen-5, killed, and processed for antigen presentation by human dendritic cells. J Immunol. 2001;**166**(2):1049-1056. DOI: 10.4049/jimmunol.166.2.1049

[50] Thind SK, Taborda CP, Nosanchuk JD. Dendritic cell interactions with Histoplasma and Paracoccidioides. Virulence. 2015;**6**(5):424-432. DOI: 10.4161/21505594.2014.965586 Epub 2015 May

[51] Mittal J, Ponce MG, Gendlina I, Nosanchuk JD. Histoplasma Capsulatum: Mechanisms for pathogenesis. Curr Top Microbiol Immunol. 2019;**422**:157-191. DOI: 10.1007/82_2018_114

[52] Williams DM, Graybill JR, Drutz DJ. Histoplasma capsulatum infection in nude mice. Infect. Immun. 1978;**21**(3):973-977

[53] Deepe GS Jr, Seder RA. Molecular and cellular determinants of immunity to Histoplasma capsulatum. Res Immunol. 1998;**149**:397-406

[54] Sharma J, Mudalagiriyappa S, Nanjappa SG. T cell responses to control fungal infection in an immunological memory lens. Front Immunol. 2022;**13**:905867

[55] Ruegg CL, Engleman EG. Impaired immunity in AIDS. The mechanisms responsible and their potential reversal by antiviral therapy. Ann N Y Acad Sci. 1990;**616**:307-317

[56] Vijayan KKV, Karthigeyan KP, Tripathi SP, Hanna LE. Pathophysiology of CD4+ T-cell depletion in HIV-1 and HIV-2 infections. Front Immunol. 2017;**8**:580

[57] Gulzar N, Copeland KFT. CD8+ T-cells: Function and response to HIV infection. Curr HIV Res. 2004;**2**(1):23-37

[58] Koppensteiner H, Brack-Werner R, Michael SM. Macrophages and their relevance in human immunodeficiency virus type I infection. Retrovirology. 2012;**9**:82

[59] Porta A, Marcsca B. Host response and Histoplasma capsulatum/macrophage molecular interactions. Medical Mycology. 2000;**38**:399-406

[60] Drak Alsibai K, Couppie P, Blanchet D, Adenis A, Epelboin L,

Blaizot R, et al. Cytological and histopathological Spectrum of histoplasmosis: 15 years of experience in French Guiana. Front. Cell. Infect. Microbiol. 2020;**10**:591974. DOI: 10.3389/fcimb.2020.591974

[61] Couppié P, Herceg K, Bourne-Watrin M, et al. The broad clinical Spectrum of disseminated histoplasmosis in HIV-infected patients: A 30 years' experience in French Guiana. J. Fungi. 2019;**5**:115. DOI: 10.3390/jof5040115

[62] Sobel JD, Vazquez JA. In: Sobel JD, Vazquez JA, editors. Contemporary Diagnosis and Management of Fungal Infections. Second ed. Handbooks in Health Care Company; 2007

[63] Kauffman CA. Histoplasmosis: A clinical and laboratory update. Clin Microbiol Rev. 2007;**20**(1):115-132. DOI: 10.1128/CMR.00027-06

[64] Tobón AM, Agudelo CA, Rosero DS, Ochoa JE, De Bedout C, Zuluaga A, et al. Disseminated histoplasmosis: A comparative study between patients with acquired immunodeficiency syndrome and non-human immunodeficiency virus-infected individuals. Am J Trop Med Hyg. 2005;**73**(3):576-582

[65] Nyalakonda H, Albuerne M, Suazo Hernandez LP, Sarria JC. Central nervous system histoplasmosis in acquired immunodeficiency syndrome. Am J Med Sci. 2016;**351**(2):177-186. DOI: 10.1016/j.amjms.2015.11.016

[66] Psarros G, Kauffman CA. Colonic histoplasmosis: A difficult diagnostic problem. Gastroenterol Hepatol (N Y). 2007;**3**(6):461-463

[67] Assi M, McKinsey DS, Driks MR, O'Connor MC, Bonacini M, Graham B, et al. Gastrointestinal histoplasmosis in the acquired immunodeficiency syndrome: Report of 18 cases and literature review. Diagn Microbiol Infect Dis. 2006;**55**(3):195-201. DOI: 10.1016/j.diagmicrobio.2006.01.015 Epub 2006 Mar 20

[68] Lamps LW, Molina CP, West AB, Haggitt RC, Scott MA. The pathologic spectrum of gastrointestinal and hepatic histoplasmosis. Am J Clin Pathol. 2000;**113**(1):64-72. DOI: 10.1309/X0Y2-P3GY-TWE8-DM02

[69] Wheat LJ, Musial CE, Jenny-Avital E. Diagnosis and management of central nervous system histoplasmosis. Clin Infect Dis. 2005;**40**(6):844-852. DOI: 10.1086/427880 Epub 2005 Feb 16

[70] Cunto MS, Corti M, Maiolo E, Santiso G, Messina F. Central nervous system involvement in patients with AIDS-associated histoplasmosis. Lung, Pulmonary & Respiratory Research Journal. 2020;**3**(1):122

[71] Azizirad O, Clifford DB, Groger RK, Prelutsky D, Schmidt RE. Histoplasmoma: Isolated central nervous system infection with Histoplasma capsulatum in a patient with AIDS. Case report and brief review of the literature. Clinical Neurology and Neurosurgery. 2007;**109**(2):176-181. DOI: 10.1016/j.clineuro.2006.04.010

[72] Wheat LJ. Diagnosis and management of histoplasmosis. Eur. J. Clin. Microbiol. Infect. Dis. 1989;**8**:480-490. DOI: 10.1007/BF01964063

[73] Nacher M, Alsibai KD, Valdes A, et al. HIV-associated disseminated histoplasmosis and rare adrenal involvement: Evidence of absence or absence of evidence. Front. Cell. Infect. Microbiol. 2021;**11**:619459

[74] Sayeed M, Benzamin M, Nahar L, Rana M, Aishy AS. Hepatic histoplasmosis:

An update. J Clin Transl Hepatol. 2022;**10**(4):726-729. DOI: 10.14218/JCTH.2020.00080 Epub 2021 Sep 22

[75] Melzani A, Reyna d, de Saint Michel R, Ntab B, et al. Incidence and trends in immune reconstitution inflammatory syndrome associated with Histoplasma capsulatum among people living with human immunodeficiency virus: A 20-year case series and literature review. Clinical Infectious Diseases. 2020;**70**(4):643-652. DOI: 10.1093/cid/ciz247

[76] Manzardo C, Guardo AC, Letang E, et al. Opportunistic infections and immune reconstitution inflammatory syndrome in HIV-1-infected adults in the combined antiretroviral therapy era: A comprehensive review. Expert Review of Anti-infective Therapy. 2015;**13**(6):751-767. DOI: 10.1586/14787210.2015.1029917

[77] Caceres DH, Tobón ÁM, Restrepo Á, Chiller T, Gómez BL. The important role of co-infections in patients with AIDS and progressive disseminated histoplasmosis (PDH): A cohort from Colombia. Med Mycol Case Rep. 2018;**19**:41-44. DOI: 10.1016/j.mmcr.2017.07.004

[78] Agudelo CA, Restrepo CA, Molina DA, et al. Tuberculosis and histoplasmosis co-infection in AIDS patients. Am J Trop Med Hyg. 2012;**87**(6):1094-1098. DOI: 10.4269/ajtmh.2012.12-0292 Epub 2012 Nov 5

[79] Caceres DH, Valdes A. Histoplasmosis and tuberculosis Co-occurrence in people with advanced HIV. J Fungi (Basel). 2019;**5**(3):73. DOI: 10.3390/jof5030073

[80] Kuate MPN, Ekeng BE, Kwizera R, Mandengue C, Bongomin F. Histoplasmosis overlapping with HIV and tuberculosis in sub-Saharan Africa: Challenges and research priorities. Ther Adv Infect Dis. 2021;**8**. DOI: 10.1177/20499361211008675

[81] Carreto-binaghi LE, Morales-villarreal FR, Garcia-de la Torre G, et al. Histoplasma capsulatum and pneumocystis jirovecii coinfection in hospitalized HIV and non-HIV patients from a tertiary care hospital in Mexico. Int J Infect Dis. 2019;**86**:65-72. DOI: 10.1016/j.ijid.2019.06.010

[82] Arias Ramos D, Alzate JA, Rico Gallego JA, Acevedo EN. Cryptococcal fungemia and probable histoplasmosis in a patient infected with HIV. Case report. BMC Infect Dis. 2018;**18**(1):704. DOI: 10.1186/s12879-018-3622-7

[83] Farooq HZ, Arfeen F, Davies C, Ahmad S, Ajdukiewicz KMB. Disseminated histoplasmosis complicated by concurrent opportunistic infections in a person living with HIV (PLHIV) — The need for infectious disease high dependency units in the United Kingdom. Clinical Infection in Practice Volumes. 2020;**3-4**:100014. DOI: 10.1016/j.clinpr.2020.100014

[84] Connolly PA, Durkin MM, Lemonte AM, Hackett EJ, Wheat LJ. Detection of histoplasma antigen by a quantitative enzyme immunoassay. Clin Vaccine Immunol. 2007;**14**(12):1587-1591. DOI: 10.1128/CVI.00071-07 Epub 2007 Oct 3

[85] Wheat LJ, Cloud G, Johnson PC, Connolly P, Goldman M, Le Monte A, et al. AIDS Clinical Trials Group; mycoses study group of NIAID. Clearance of fungal burden during treatment of disseminated histoplasmosis with liposomal amphotericin B versus itraconazole. Antimicrob Agents Chemother. 2001;**45**(8):2354-2357. DOI: 10.1128/AAC.45.8.2354-2357.2001

[86] Wheat LJ, Connolly-Stringfield P, Blair R, Connolly K, Garringer T, Katz BP.

Histoplasmosis relapse in patients with AIDS: Detection using Histoplasma capsulatum variety capsulatum antigen levels. Ann Intern Med. 1991;**115**(12):936-941. DOI: 10.7326/0003-4819-115-12-936

[87] Wheat J, Myint T, Guo Y, Kemmer P, Hage C, Terry C, et al. Central nervous system histoplasmosis: Multicenter retrospective study on clinical features, diagnostic approach and outcome of treatment. Medicine (Baltimore). 2018;**97**(13):e0245. DOI: 10.1097/MD.0000000000010245 Erratum in: Medicine (Baltimore). 2018;97(16):e0537

[88] Huber F, Nacher M, Aznar C, Pierre-Demar M, El Guedj M, Vaz T, et al. AIDS-related Histoplasma capsulatum var. capsulatum infection: 25 years experience of French Guiana. AIDS. 2008;**22**(9):1047-1053. DOI: 10.1097/QAD.0b013e3282ffde67

[89] Kirn DH, Fredericks D, McCutchan JA, Stites D, Shuman M. Serum ferritin levels correlate with disease activity in patients with AIDS and disseminated histoplasmosis. Clin Infect Dis. 1995;**21**(4):1048-1049. DOI: 10.1093/clinids/21.4.1048

[90] Daher EF, Silva GB Jr, Barros FA, Takeda CF, Mota RM, Ferreira MT, et al. Clinical and laboratory features of disseminated histoplasmosis in HIV patients from Brazil. Trop Med Int Health. 2007;**12**:1108-1115

[91] Wheat LJ, Freifeld AG, Kleiman MB, et al. Clinical practice guidelines for the management of patients with histoplasmosis: 2007 update by the Infectious Diseases Society of America. Clin Infect Dis. 2007;**45**(7):807-825. DOI: 10.1086/521259

[92] Johnson PC, Wheat LJ, Cloud GA, Goldman M, Lancaster D, Bamberger DM, et al. National Institute of Allergy and Infectious Diseases mycoses study group. Safety and efficacy of liposomal amphotericin B compared with conventional amphotericin B for induction therapy of histoplasmosis in patients with AIDS. Ann Intern Med. 2002;**137**(2):105-109. DOI: 10.7326/0003-4819-137-2-200207160-00008

[93] Panel on Guidelines for the Prevention and Treatment of Opportunistic Infections in Adults and Adolescents with HIV. Guidelines for the Prevention and Treatment of Opportunistic Infections in Adults and Adolescents with HIV. National Institutes of Health, Centers for Disease Control and Prevention, HIV Medicine Association and Infectious Diseases Society of America. Available at: https://clinicalinfo.hiv.gov/en/guidelines/adult-and-adolescent-opportunistic-infection. [Accessed 07MAR2023] [page O-1-5]

[94] Andes D, Pascual A, Marchetti O. Antifungal therapeutic drug monitoring: Established and emerging indications. Antimicrob Agents Chemother. 2009;**53**(1):24-34. DOI: 10.1128/AAC.00705-08 Epub 2008 Oct 27

[95] University of Liverpool, HIV Drug Interaction. Available from: https://www.hiv-druginteractions.org

[96] Restrepo A, Tobón A, Clark B, Graham DR, Corcoran G, Bradsher RW, et al. Salvage treatment of histoplasmosis with posaconazole. J Infect. 2007;**54**(4):319-327. DOI: 10.1016/j.jinf.2006.05.006 Epub 2006 Jul 7

[97] Gonçalves D, Ferraz C, Vaz L. Posaconazole as rescue therapy in African histoplasmosis. Braz J Infect Dis. 2013;**17**(1):102-105. DOI: 10.1016/j.bjid.2012.06.027 Epub 2013 Jan 9

[98] Wheat LJ, Connolly P, Haddad N, Le Monte A, Brizendine E, Hafner R.

Antigen clearance during treatment of disseminated histoplasmosis with itraconazole versus fluconazole in patients with AIDS. Antimicrob. Agents Chemother. 2002;**46**:248-250. DOI: 10.1128/AAC.46.1.248-250.2002

[99] McKinsey DS. Treatment and prevention of histoplasmosis in adults living with HIV. J Fungi (Basel). 2021;7(6):429. DOI: 10.3390/jof7060429

[100] Murray M, Hine P. Treating progressive disseminated histoplasmosis in people living with HIV. Cochrane Database Syst. Rev. 2020;**4**:CD013594

[101] Hendrix MJ, Larson L, Rauseo AM, Rutjanawech S, Franklin AD, Powderly WG, et al. Voriconazole versus Itraconazole for the initial and step-down treatment of histoplasmosis: A retrospective cohort. Clin Infect Dis. 2021;**73**(11):e3727-e3732. DOI: 10.1093/cid/ciaa1555

[102] Mazzella A, Stone NRH, Pool ERM, García Mingo A, Bolache S, Wood C. HIV-associated disseminated histoplasmosis successfully treated with isavuconazole consolidation therapy. Med Mycol Case Rep. 2019;**27**:42-43. DOI: 10.1016/j.mmcr.2019.12.013

[103] McKinsey DS, Wheat LJ, Cloud GA, Pierce M, Black JR, Bamberger DM, et al. National Institute of Allergy and Infectious Diseases Mycoses Study Group. Itraconazole prophylaxis for fungal infections in patients with advanced human immunodeficiency virus infection: Randomized, placebo-controlled, double-blind study. Clin Infect Dis. 1999;**28**(5):1049-1056. DOI: 10.1086/514744